Benjamin Ward Richardson

On Alcohol

A Course of Six Cantor Lectures Delivered Before the Society of Arts

Benjamin Ward Richardson

On Alcohol
A Course of Six Cantor Lectures Delivered Before the Society of Arts

ISBN/EAN: 9783744669962

Printed in Europe, USA, Canada, Australia, Japan

Cover: Foto ©ninafisch / pixelio.de

More available books at **www.hansebooks.com**

ON

ALCOHOL:

*A COURSE OF SIX CANTOR LECTURES DELIV-
ERED BEFORE THE SOCIETY OF ARTS.*

BY

BENJAMIN W. RICHARDSON, M.A., M.D., F.R.S.,

FELLOW OF THE ROYAL COLLEGE OF PHYSICIANS, AND HONORARY
PHYSICIAN TO THE ROYAL LITERARY FUND.

NEW YORK:

The National Temperance Society and Publication House,

58 READE STREET.

—

1876.

INTRODUCTORY NOTE.

THE course of Cantor Lectures on Alcohol here published were prepared at the request of the Council of the Society of Arts, and were delivered before the Society in the months of November, December, January, and February last.

I do not remember to have delivered any Lectures that have attracted so much earnest public attention, and in publishing them in this cheap form I am responding to a request too general to admit of hesitation or delay on my part. With the exception of the transference of the tabular matter into an Appendix, the introduction of a few minor and verbal corrections, and the addition of a page of learned and interesting passages kindly communicated to me by Mr. Stanford, M.A., F.R.S., the Lectures are published as they were spoken.

In this form I found them favorably received by the large audiences who honored me with their attention, and I am, therefore, led to hope for them equal favor with the larger public to whom they are now addressed.

It remains for me only to add, that though I have spoken out freely the lessons I have learned from nature, no pledge binds me, and no society banded to propagate particular views and tenets claims my allegiance. I stand forth simply as an interpreter of natural fact and law.

12 HINDE STREET, W.
May 1, 1875.

CONTENTS

V.

VI.

PREFACE.

I AM very glad to learn that the "Course of Cantor Lectures on Alcohol," delivered by B. W. Richardson, M.D., F.R.S., before the Edinburgh Society of Arts, is about to be presented to the American public. They are clear, scientific, and couched in language free from technicalities and easily understood by all. I have seen no work on this subject so satisfactory as these lectures, which present it without "special pleading"; I hope they will be carefully read in every household. Aiming as they do to impart knowledge based on sound scientific principles, to the public mind, they cannot fail to awaken it to a realization of the evil that is being wrought by this agency, most destructive to human life and usefulness.

Alcohol has no place in the healthy system, but is an "irritant poison," producing a diseased condition of body and mind. Statistics show that ten per cent. of the annual number of deaths in this country are due to alcohol; that fully thirty-five per cent. of our insane, are so either directly or indirectly from its use; and that from seventy-five to ninety per cent. of the inmates of our penal and pauper institutions owe their condition to its influence. Besides this, we find that forty-five per cent. of the inmates of our asylums for idiots, are the offspring of parents addicted to drink.

Destroying as its use does, the will, the judgment, and the moral sense, may we not with propriety consider it a cause of that low state of public and private integrity which permits, even in our very midst, the formation of those shameful combinations to defraud and steal commonly known as "rings"?

Now the question meets us, how can this destruction of lives valuable to the state in their productiveness, be arrested, and a better condition of things be brought about, so that the burden of our taxation be lightened—taxation of which the great proportion goes to support our drinking-classes and their off-spring. Let public intelligence and public morals be so educated that the *cause* of these things be appreciated, and so appreciated that they shall insist on laying the axe at the root of the tree, instead of lopping off the branches, by *preventing* a traffic in alcohol, instead of punishing the unfortunate victims of its use.

In Pennsylvania, in the year 1867, for every fourteen dollars received from license fees, the State expended one hundred in the support of the victims of alcohol; on principles of political economy, is this sound legislation?

If the habitual use of distilled liquors increase as rapidly within the opening century as it has during the one just ending, how sad the outlook! I can discern nothing in the future but a wreck of national honor, and the sinking to a lower standard of civilization and morality, unless public sentiment in this regard be changed. As a means to this end, let me again express the hope that these lectures may be carefully read in every home in the land.

WILLARD PARKER, M.D., etc.

ON ALCOHOL.

LECTURE I.

ON ALCOHOL, IN RELATION TO SOME OF ITS VARIED
SERVICES TO MANKIND.

WE had before us a few weeks since an interesting national event. It was that of an archbishop and a minister of the Crown speaking almost at the same time, on one of the most important subjects of the day, viz., the part performed by alcohol on the national stage as it is set forth and played upon at this period of our history. The distinguished prelate took naturally for his view of the subject the moral influence of alcohol, and from this point denounced alcohol, in whatever form it presents itself for human consumption, in terms as eloquent as they were persuasive and forcible. The statesman took for his view of the subject the financial influence of alcohol; he gave a clear and by no means exaggerated estimate of the importance of an agent which, in these kingdoms, rests on an invested capital of not less than one hundred

13

and seventeen millions of money ; and submitted, in conclusive terms, an argument, which, contrasted with that of the prelate, means that an agent so commercially potential cannot be materially interfered with in the present stage of our civilization, whatever may be the result of its influence on the community for good or for evil.

To the utterances of the church and of the legislative chamber we are accustomed to listen with such regard, that when any representative of either body speaks, we turn an ear almost automatically, and accept what is said as commanding respect, even though we dissent from the opinions that are expressed. No one therefore who stands out of these spheres can hope to obtain a hearing extended so far and wide, and equally authoritative.

And yet there is scope for honest utterance on another side of the alcohol question. The prelate and the legislator can hardly have more intimate conversance with the influence of alcohol than the physician and man of science. To the moral view of the question and to the legislative may well therefore be added the physical, and it is to this I shall try to direct public attention in these discourses, conscious, fully, of the disadvantages under which I should labor were it not for the countenance and support I shall hope to receive from you.

The strain running through all these lectures, in however diverse a manner the subject-matter of them may be pursued, will then be simply this : Of what physical value has alcohol been to man ?

of what value is it to man? We know it is of no
value to any other animal, and thus we limit our
inquiry at once to the highest order of the ani-
mate series of natural development, or of natural
creation.

In the studies that are in this sense to be under-
taken, I will not fail to remember the injunction
placed upon me to speak simply and plainly; not
to offend pride of learning by too great simplicity
of statement, nor yet to embarrass humility by a
display of technical language and of the abstruse
technical reasoning, for which the subject in hand
affords so much opportunity. As far as possible I
will strive to be plainness itself, and that, not only
in mode of expression, but in matter of it; I mean
in truthfulness of expression, as far as I am guided
by the light that enables me to see what is nearest
to the truth.

I shall propose in this description to glance first
at the value of alcohol to man in a general sense;
that is to say, to its value as an agent useful for
other purposes than as a fluid to be imbibed. From
this I shall be naturally led to consider its action,
physically, on man, and its use as a fluid consumed
with, and, according to common acceptation, as a
food. Lastly, I shall be brought to treat upon its
secondary action on the vital functions, physical
and mental, i.e., on the deteriorations of structure
and derangements of function, which may follow
its use.

THE TERM "ALCOHOL."

The first employment of the word alcohol is obscurely recorded.　Bartholomew Parr, one of the most learned of our scientific classics, taking the usual derivation of the word as from the Arabic *A'l-ka-hol*, a subtile essence, says it was originally employed to designate an impalpable powder, used by the Eastern women to tinge the hair and the margins of the eyelids.　As this powder, viz., an ore of lead, was impalpable, the same name was given to other subtile powders, and then to the spirit of wine exalted to its highest purity and perfection.

The earliest systematic and truly scientific use of the term that I can discover is in Nicholas Lemert's 'Course of Chemistry,' published in 1698. There the word is used as a verb, " to alcoholize," and the definition of this is said to be " to reduce to alcohol, as when a mixture is beaten into an impalpable powder."　The word, says Lemert, is also used to express a very fine spirit ; " thus the spirit of wine well rectified is called the alcohol of wine."

The word employed in this sense merely tells us of a refined fluid substance obtained by a subtile process of separation from a grosser substance. But it was not applied to the special fluid now under our consideration until long after that fluid had actually been separated.　Then it was used as a supplementary term to the earlier terms, *Vinum adustum, Vinum ardens, Spiritus vini, Spiritus ardens,* by which a spirit obtained from the grosser fluid, by the action of fire, was known and described.

FERMENTATION OF WINE.

We must now go back to a much earlier study, viz., to the study of the primitive fluid, from which the subtile spirit was derived. In the history of the production of alcohol we gather, in fact, the use of two of the most prominent words of our modern language : fermentation and distillation. They each mark distinct progressive epochs in natural science.

The term fermentation brings us in contact with the primitive fluid. It leads us to ask how, from the vegetable world, by change or mutation of its matter, a new product was evolved? The origin of this procedure is so old we have no possible means of tracing it. Before ever the word chemistry, or the science which that word implies, was dreamed of, this process of obtaining the crude liquor, from which alcohol was ultimately extracted, was in active operation. By some accidental discovery it had been started by human hands, and the act of first lighting and reproducing fire was hardly a less wonderful development of the higher faculties resident in man, than was this discovery. The operation itself, originally, was, we may presume, very simple. As there is a spontaneity in nature to produce fire, as for instance, when a metal like iron strikes a stone, so there is a spontaneity of fermentation in vegetable matter—especially in the juices of fresh ripe fruits in warm weather—which fact being observed, first, from the motion induced in the fluids, and secondly from the crude products that were left, would lead naturally to the contemplation of the steps of the process, to its easy, artificial, and more perfect development, to a method of separating and purifying the products, and afterwards of tasting and using them.

The products of fermenting fruits were limited to four : an active air which escapes freely ; a froth or yeast which floats above as a crust ; a heavy mass or lees which sinks to the bottom ; and a fluid which remains apart. These portions, each readily separable, indeed, separable of themselves, were soon understood in respect of their virtues. That invisible air, which escapes so actively, is a deadly vapor or miasm ; that froth, unpleasant to the taste, is an active promoter of the motion that springs from the fruit ; those lees are like sediment from muddy water, excrementitious, to be cast away ; but that remaining subtile fluid, to the palate so grateful, to the senses so exhilarating, to the heart so forcing, to the intellect so exciting or so deadening :—let it be brought forth in the daintiest cups the handicrafts can fashion from the rude earth ! It is not, to the savage, a mortal thing at all. Water flows in open streams, a common liquid, at which cattle and creeping things may drink ; this must be the drink of the superior intelligences from whom the savage came ! It lifts the man who takes it into a higher sphere of life, or it degrades him to the lowest. It introduces him, as it were, to a new human organization that is not to be a passing phenomenon, but, for good or for evil, is to remain for ages.

The fluid is wine.

The discovery is an epoch surpassed by none

other, in the history of one portion of mankind, and the early dawning civilizations show
their wonder at it in their mythology. Egypt
claims the invention for her god Osiris, Greece for
Bacchus, and Rome for Saturn. The Greeks, most
ambitious to be connected with the origin, assert
that the very name belongs to them, for the drink
was first discovered in Ætolia by Orestheus, the
son of Deucalion, whose grandson, Oeneus, was so
called from Oinos, which was the old name of the
vine. Or else the discovery was by Oeneus himself, who first pressed the rich grapes. Thus
Oinos—oinon—vinum—wine. Then by these nations the praises of wine and of the wine gods, one
and all, were sung into the later times. The first
of the Roman poets, excited to his labor by Mæce-
nas, the friend of Augustus, who would that the
vineyards should flourish, is thus prompted to in-
voke Bacchus, under the name of Pater Lenæus—

> " Hither, oh, Lenæus—Father Lenæus, come.
> By thee with heavy viny harvest crowned,
> The pasture flourishes. In the full vats
> The vintage foams.
> Hither Lenæus, Father Lenæus come,
> And, with thy buskins off, in the new wine,
> Stain, thou, thy naked legs even with me."

And thus on until our own era, in which—alas for
the mutability of even god-like virtues!—under
the title of " The Worship of Bacchus," our veteran artist, George Cruikshank, has turned the
praises of his brother artist, Virgil, into scorn, and
has transformed Pater Lenæus the wine giver,

into the destroyer of every civilization over which he has become enthroned.

It is worthy here of special remark that the invention of wine was local on the planet, and that it came from some centre of the ancient world lying near to those points from whence our modern civilization took its rise. For when that civilization concentrated itself into bands or armies, or navies, for the purpose of discovering new portions of the earth, where other savage nations, as they are called, dwell, it found the wine god, the wine cup, and the wine equally unknown. A good three-quarters of the old world knew no more of wine than of the people who invented it, until they were taught to know it—then they learned about it fast enough.

The practice of exciting fermentation and of obtaining the coveted fermented liquor once known, the knowledge was extended, until from varied vegetable substances wine became a product extracted by an art that was successful, however rude. The discovery of the ferment, that is to say of the body that would produce fermentation, was sufficient to set in mutation or intestine motion a whole series of fermentable vegetable substances, and to extend the manufacture of various vinous fluids to an unlimited degree. From the expressed juice of the grape the transition was easy to other juicy fruits, such as the mulberry, the apple, the pear, the peach: from these again to those juices which exude from trees, as from the Eastern palm-tree; and from these again to such similar looking substances as manna and honey. From fruits, moreover, it was an easy transition to seeds, and from seeds that were soft and succulent to seeds that were hard and of the character of what we now call grain.

From all these varied sources of fermentable substances there was produced for ages the fluid containing the basis of alcohol. Its most common name was wine, though the term was modified by adjective additions signifying sometimes its color, sometimes the place where it was made or marketed. Thus were introduced the white and red wines, the Vino Tinto and the golden unctuous Vino Greco. Even after the discovery (of which I shall soon again speak) of the existence of a distinct essence or spirit in wine, the original fluid held pre-eminence over all other strong drinks, and in the early and middle stages of civilization in Europe the number of wines that were used exceeded anything we now have in common use. In the Appendix to these lectures, there will be found, in a table—Table I.—lists of ancient Roman wines arranged in nine groups.

As a matter of some historical interest, it is worth a moment or two to touch on the special qualities of a few of those vinous drinks.

Certain of the ancient Roman wines of the first group were home wines. The Falernian, one of these, was, it is believed, something like our modern Madeira, and was not commonly used until it was ten years old. After it was twenty years old it affected the body unfavorably, causing headache. This was the experience of Galen.

Other wines were foreign. Chian, also called

the Ariusian, of which there were three varieties—
austere, sweet, and intermediate—and the Lesbian,
considered to be a diuretic, were of this kind.

Some wines were named after their color, as
white, dark, and red. The white were thought to
be the thinnest and least heating ; the dark-colored
and sweet the most nourishing ; the red the most
heating.

Some, again, were named after qualities, of age,
and the like : as old (Vetus); new (Novum); of the
present year (Hornum); of three years (Trimum);
mellow (Molle, Lene, Vetustate edentulum); rough
(Asperum); pure (Merum); strong (Fortius).

Certain wines, named Myndian, Halicarnassian,
Rhodian, and Coan, were made with salt water.
They were considered not to be intoxicating, but
to promote digestion.

Two wines, Cnidian and Adrian, were also medicinal wines. The first, it was believed, engendered blood and was at the same time a laxative ;
the second was diaphoretic.

Mustum was a term applied to wine newly made,
or the fresh juice of the grape. Protropum was the
juice which runs from the grapes without pressing.
Mulsum was a mixture of wine and honey. Sapa
was Mustum boiled down to a third. Defrutum
was Mustum reduced to half, and Carenum was
the same reduced to a third.

Passum was a sweet wine, prepared from grapes
that had been dried in the sun. Passum creticum,
also a sweet wine, is believed to have been the same
as the wine which our own forefathers called Malmsey; the wine in which the Duke of Clarence

brother of Edward the Fourth, elected to be drowned.

A wine called Murrhina, placed in the last group in the Appendix, has a curious history. The Greeks had a wine of this kind, which consisted of pure wine perfumed with odorous substances. The Romans had a wine similarly named, which is supposed to have been wine mingled with myrrh. It was administered to those who were about to suffer torture, in order to intoxicate them and to remove the sense of suffering.

The ancient wines retained their place probably until the end of the Middle Ages, but we have no reliable evidence bearing upon this point, if we except an occasional reference by some poet or physician to the subject of wine. Very slowly the names, rather than the wines, changed generally. The Roman conqueror who built his villa on our islands, and fitted it with so much taste and means of luxury, added to it his wine-cellar, in the manner he had been instructed by his forefathers, and from it took out his red and white and old wine, as we do now; boasting possibly of the vintage from which it was grown, and eloquent as to its age and perfect ripeness. If he had no old port, he had old Falernian or Passum; his rough and his sweet, his light and his heavy wines, the same as our connoisseur of to-day. But, perhaps, he knew a great deal more, in the way of fact about the vintages, than his modern follower.

How the wines changed in name through the centuries will be gathered from the lists of the wines of Europe in use in the last century, collected

by the distinguished chemist Neumann, and detail-
ed in the Appendix, Table II.

Some of the wines mediæval and later derive additional names from peculiarities in themselves.
Sec, from which we derive the name of the wine
Sack, on which Sir John Falstaff so keenly enjoyed
himself, means dry ; the wine being made from half
dried grapes. Malmsey was called by the Italians
" Manna alla bocca e balsamo al cervello "—" Manna to the mouth and balsam to the brain."

From the chemist of last century, Neumann, who
has collected for us such a long list of wines, we
are supplied with a very instructive table of analyses showing the amount of spirit present in the
different specimens. The wines he analysed are
tabulated in alphabetical order. I believe his to
be the first true chemical analyses that were ever
made, on an extensive and comparative scale, of
different wines, and if they indicate all the spirit in
the wines named, it is clear that the amount of
spirit in them was exceedingly small, when compared with what is present in the wines of the
present day. Malmsey, the strongest of them, contained but about twelve per cent. of spirit, and
sack a little more than half that amount. Falstaff
might readily drink at a draught a pint of sack
that contained rather less than seven and a half
per cent. of spirit.

BEER.

The only other diluted rival of wine obtained
by fermentation was the liquid derived from corn.
Tradition, active again in giving celestial origin

to strong drinks, has assigned the introduction of the art of making this product first to Osiris, the divinity of Egypt, and afterwards to the goddess Ceres. The fluid thus produced became, in Saxon language, known as beer, bere, from barley, or perhaps from the Hebrew, *bar*, corn. Tacitus calls it Zythum. The Egyptians, it is said, made it first for the common folk that they too might receive the gift of Osiris. In its original state beer was what we would now call the sweet fluid or wort fresh from the vat, and untinctured with any additional substance. So it continued probably until the ninth century, when it began to be treated with the *lupulus*, or hop. The first mention of this plant is made by an Arabian, named Mesue, of about the year 850, but he does not refer to it in relation to beer. The hop not only flavored but tended to preserve the beer, and in a few centuries it became of general use. In the reign of Henry the Sixth the use of hops was for a time forbidden, on the ground that they spoiled the beer and rendered it dangerous. An order prohibiting hops and sulphur for beer was also made in the reign of Henry the Eighth. But the hops at last won their way. It is worthy of notice that Neumann, who analysed the beers of last century, as well as the wines, found that the beers contained an amount of spirit varying from 5 per cent. in the weakest, to 10.90 per cent. in the strongest kinds. The malt liquors of the last century were, it appears from this, of much the same strength as those of the present.

Thus in the history of alcohol the first step of

discovery was that of its production from vegetable matter by the process of fermentation. As so produced it was a mixture of that which we now call pure spirit, or alcohol, with water, and with small quantities of other extraneous substances of minor moment.

On the nature of the fermentative change by which the juice of the fruit, or the exuded fluid of the plant or tree, or the seed or the sweet sugar, is transformed into the new product, speculation has been rife for a hundred years at least. In this day the atomic constitution of water, of alcohol, and of the substances which yield alcohol are known, and the atomic change of constitution that takes place is known; but the reason of the process is, according to my judgment, as little understood as it was when the discussion began. Probably, indeed, the latest theories that have been advanced are rather a retrogression, by a line of learned subtleties, from the earlier views, than an approach to simplicity of truth. I do not, therefore, venture to trouble you with any description on this head. One word I would add in the way of a guard against misuse of terms from assumed analogies. We often hear processes described as fermentative, which in truth have no relation, by any proved physical argument, with the true process of fermentation of vegetable matter connected with the production of wine. To take one example; we speak commonly of the zymotic or fermentative diseases, applying the term to those maladies which, in the form of contagious fevers, become epidemic. Hence many are led to believe that in these diseases there is in the body an actual fermentation like that in wine or beer; a comparison no closer, according to our knowledge as it now actually exists, than might be instituted between the same process and the so called ferment of a mob when it assembles to give vent to its turbulent rage.

DISTILLATION.

I have said that for many centuries there was nothing known to mankind beyond the formation of a vinous fluid. At length a new process was brought to bear on wine, which simple as it is to us now, was in its early days, and for many long days afterwards, a wonder and a mystery. This was the simple act of distilling wine, and of obtaining from it by distillation a fine spirit containing no water. The discovery of distillation of wine has been attributed to Albucasis, or Casa, an Arabian chemist and physician of the eleventh century. The evidence on this point is not very convincing. It is true that the refined body called spirit of wine began to be known in alchemical and Arabian schools about or soon after the time of Casa, and from that circumstance, rather than from direct evidence derived from his works, the discovery has probably been imputed to him. However, it is historically correct that from the school of Albucasis the discovery sprang. The alchemists or adepts were conversant with pure spirit, and, says Boerhaave, when they had reduced it to the utmost subtlety, they made use of it in the preparations of all their secret menstruums.

Distillation itself was probably an imitation of
nature, for nature is ever distilling and condensing. In the cold, water condenses on the leaf and
on the grass, as dew, and ascends as vapor in the
sun. This process of raising water into a state of
vapor by heat, and condensing it by cold, the
simplest of immediate imitations of nature, would
by easy transition pass to other liquids, and with
special ease to that liquid which has rivalled water
as a drink for man—wine.

The pure spirit of wine in its earlier use was
applied mainly to chemical and medicinal purposes, and indeed many centuries elapsed before
the process of distillation became active for the
production of those stronger drinks, which, under
the name of "spirits," are now in such common
use in daily life. Brandy from *brennen*, to burn ;
thus *Branntwein*, brandy, is a comparatively late
term in European literature. Gin, contracted
from Geneva, is not to be found as signifying a
spirituous drink in our vocabularies of two hundred years ago. The term rum is assigned to the
native American peoples, who so designated the
vinous spirit distilled from sugar ; and whiskey
(Celtic *uisge*, water), though it · may have been
known as a distilled drink as long as Branntwein,
has not been Anglicised, I believe, for more than
a century and a half. Some further notes on this
subject by Mr. Stanford will be found in the Appendix.

In the earlier modes of distillation the instruments used were simple but effective. They consisted of the furnace, the receptacle to the furnace,

the receiver which stood within the receptacle, and the alembic or condenser, which was made of tin or other metal.

The ancient alembic, the use of which is still valued, was, in truth, a very scientific instrument, and caused a perfect collection of the distilled fluid. The spirit from the crude wine ascended from a heated reservoir into a conical tube, and then downwards through a returning exit tube into a receiver.

The adepts were, indeed, marvellously mechanical, and when we recall that they neither had cork nor elastic tubing, nor gas, we wonder by what clever devices they were so successful. They had many useful arts, I am sure, which we have improperly forgotten, and which might with advantage be revived. Some of their instruments, for a long time thought to be fanciful and useless, are being again considered of value. One of these was called a cohobator, and another called a circulator, in which they caused spirits to boil and distil, and condense and distil again, for months at a time. The fluids went round and round in the circulator like the wheel of fortune, and many an adept has looked upon his fortune as spinning in that wheel, from which the elixir of life and the philosopher's stone were, in his ardent imagination, to be evolved.

To sum up, let us remember the four stages in the general history of alcohol, from the first to the time when it came strictly under analytical chemical observation; and, in regard to common knowledge, to the present time.

(*a.*) The stage of manufacture of wine or beer by fermentation. A stage extending from the earliest history until the time of the adepts, say about the eleventh century of the Christian era.

(*b.*) A stage when there was distilled from the wine a lighter spirit called, first, spirit of wine, and afterwards alcohol.

(*c.*) A stage when this subtile or distilled spirit from wine was applied in its refined and pure state to the arts and to the sciences.

(*d.*) A stage when this same process of distillation was applied to the production of alcoholic spirits for the use of man as spirituous drinks, under the names of brandy, gin, whiskey, rum,—a stage comparatively modern.

USES OF WINE.

We will, if you please, leave now, for a time, the consideration of wine and alcohol as drinks, and dwell briefly on the uses to which these fluids have been applied for other purposes. The study is peculiarly interesting, and I could easily carry you on during the whole course of these lectures with the narration of it. Unfortunately every word I have to say must be introduced into this hour, so that I can refer only to the salient points, and to a few only of these.

From the first, the preservative or antiseptic quality of wine was recognised, and the fluid was employed for the preservation of animal and vegetable substances. The Roman butchers, who, like our modern butchers, sold their fresh and their salted meats, prepared their salted flesh in the following manner:—The animals they intended to preserve were kept from drinking any fluid on the eve of the day on which the killing took place. After the killing the parts to be preserved were boned and sprinkled lightly with pounded salt. Then, having well dried off all dampness, the operators sprinkled more salt, and placed the pieces so as not to touch each other, in vessels that had been used for oil or vinegar. Over the whole they poured sweet wine, covered the contents of the vessel with straw, and, when they could, kept down the temperature of the room in which the vessel was placed by sprinkling snow around. When the cook wished to remove the salt from the meat, he took it out of the wine and boiled it first in milk and afterwards in rain water.

Long previous to the Roman era this preservative process of wine had been recognised and applied. Palm wine was used by the Egyptians in their most costly processes of embalming the bodies of the dead. This same application of wine, or spirits of wine, for the preservation of animal and also of vegetable substances, has been maintained up to our time. In our museums the specimens therein preserved, in the moist state, are immersed in spirit, and the modern art of embalming is not perfected without the employment of the same antiseptic agent.

Early after the discovery of the properties of wine the fact must have been observed that from a change in it another substance was produced, to which, in these days, we give the name of vinegar.

To prevent the formation of vinegar in wine, the ancients boiled the wine, and to remove the acidity arising from vinegar they added gypsum to sour wine, and thus rendered it palatable. Vinegar itself they employed for purposes precisely the same as we in this day; they partook of it with vegetables, they employed it for preservation of animal and vegetable substances, and they applied it for numerous medicinal purposes. After the process of distillation was discovered by the adepts, the distillation of vinegar was also carried on, and in this way was obtained that strong vinegar, which enters so largely into various uses as an acid, called aromatic vinegar.

Very early in history wine was employed for another purpose, that, namely, of extracting the active principles from plants and other substances possessing, or supposed to possess, medicinal virtues. Dioscorides, one of the fathers of medicine, and particularly of that part which pertains to the use of curative substances, or medicaments proper, is full of descriptions of vinous tinctures, some of which were sufficiently potent even for our present use. A vinous tincture of this kind has a very singular and, I had almost said, romantic history. This is the wine of Mandragora. In the Isles of Greece there has grown for ages a plant called mandrake; it belongs to the same family of plants as our belladonna, or deadly nightshade. From the root of this plant the Greeks extracted, by means of wine, a narcotic, and what in this day we should call an anæsthetic. Some, says our learned Dioscorides, boil the root in the wine down to a third part and preserve the decoction, of which they administer a cyathus (about what would now be a common wineglassful), for want of sleep, or for severe pains of any part, and also before operations with the knife or cautery, that these may not be felt. Again, he says, a wine is prepared from the bark without boiling, and three pounds of it are put into a cadus (about eighteen gallons) of sweet wine, and three cyathi of this are given to those who are cut or cauterised, when, being thrown into a deep sleep, they do not feel any pain. Again, he speaks of a preparation of mandragora called morion, which causes infatuation and takes away the reason. Under the influence of this agent the person sleeps, without sense, in the attitude in which he took it, for three or four hours afterwards. Pliny, the Roman historian, bears evidence, much later, to the same effect, and adds the singular remark that some persons have sought sleep from the smell of this medicine. And again, Lucius Apuleius, the author of the book called the 'Golden Ass,' who lived about 160 A.D., and of whose works eleven editions were republished in the fourteenth and fifteenth centuries, says that if a man has to have a limb mutilated, sawn, or burnt, he may take half an ounce of mandragora in wine, and whilst he sleeps the member may be cut off without pain or sense.

It is unquestionably to this same anæsthetic wine our own Shakespeare refers in his half-imaginary, half-legendary Middle Age history. This is the wine of that insane root, which, says Macbeth, "takes the reason prisoner." This is the

wine that Juliet drinks, and the action of which
the Friar Lawrence describes—

> "Through all thy veins shall run
> A cold and drowsy humor, which shall seize
> Each vital spirit ; for no pulse shall keep
> His natural progress, but surcease to beat :
> No warmth, no breath, shall testify thou liv'st ;
> The roses in thy lips and cheeks shall fade
> To paly ashes ; thy eyes' windows fall,
> Like death when he shuts up the day of life ;
> Each part, deprived of supple government,
> Shall stiff, and stark, and cold appear like death :
> And in this borrow'd likeness of shrunk death
> Thou shalt remain full two and forty hours,
> And then awake as from a pleasant sleep."

It follows therefore from the history of scientific
discovery that our modern great advance of removing pain during surgical operations is in fact,
if not as old as the hills, as old almost as wine.
But is the story true, you say ? I answer Yes,
and the answer is from experiment. Thinking it
a subject of very great interest, I instituted, a few
years ago, an inquiry into the matter. Through
the kindness of my friend, the late Mr. Daniel
Hanbury, F.R.S., I obtained a fine specimen of
mandragora root, and I made once again, after a
lapse of probably five centuries, Mandragora wine.
I tested this, and found it was a narcotic having
precisely the properties that were anciently ascribed to it. I found that in animals it would produce even the sleep of Juliet, not for thirty or forty
hours, a term that must be accepted as a poetical
licence, but for the four hours named by Dioscorides easily, and that in awakening there was an

excitement which tallies with the same phenomenon that was observed by the older physicians.

Thus, one of the first uses of wine to man was amongst the most noble and beneficent that man by his ingenuity can confer on his kind, and if wine had ever been used in this way and in none worse, Pater Lenæus might have retained his supremacy in the good opinion of all the world.

Besides using wine for extracting the virtues of the vegetable kingdom, our ancient chemists tested it on metals and made it here subservient to their purpose. What they called the extract of Mars was a solution of iron, made with an astringent wine, and reduced into a thick consistency by fire. Eight ounces of the rust of iron, powdered very fine, were put into an iron pot and covered with four pints of strong red wine. The iron crucible was then set on the fire, and the mixture, stirred with an iron rod, was boiled to a third: then it was strained through a cloth and evaporated into an extract. To this extract wonderful curative powers were ascribed, and indeed it was a very useful medicine. The metal antimony also was subjected to the action of wine. The so called liver of antimony was treated with white wine and dissolved in it, and to this day we retain the remedy. It was originally called the emetic wine.

USES OF SPIRIT OF WINE OR ALCOHOL.

After the process of distillation of wine was discovered, the use of the new spirit rose rapidly into application in a variety of ways. The adepts, the

Middle Age chemists of whom I have spoken, kept this distilled spirit long a secret. They found in it a solvent for many things that before were insoluble. Oils, resins, gum resins, balsams were now brought into a medium that acted towards them as a menstruum, and straightway they were dissolved. The East Indian Styrax Benzoin yielded a balsam which, dissolved in the distilled spirit, was a fortune to the chemists. The Commander's balsam, or balsam for wounds, or Friar's balsam, was soon the reputed heal-all of every injury.

The useful extracted first out of the new distillate, beauty was next remembered. Alas for the female face divine, the cosmetic and the subtile wash that should veritably make young faces old and assumably make old faces young, were soon in process in the laboratory of the adept who could distil wine. Again, the artist came in for a share in the discovery. The once insoluble and the useless resins and ambers were dissolved for his brush, and gave him coatings, preservatives, and washings, of which previously he had no conception.

This spirit of wine burns. It does not touch oil for the light it gives, but how strange! it burns away without a trace of smoke, and with an excellent heat. So the spirit lamp in due time is invented. A trifle, say you? Nay, it was as great an advance to the chemist who first used it as the gas in the Bunsen burner is to us.

Once more; this subtle spirit has in it the virtue of preserving all organic substances with which it is brought in contact. It masters putrefaction itself; perchance the elixir of life is therefore found.

It dissolves insoluble bodies; perchance it will by careful study and experiment reveal the grand secret of transmutation. In this way reasoned its first masters.

I must not dwell longer over these details of minor things of major usefulness. I must turn to some applications of our refined spirit which are major in fact as well as in use, in theory as well as in practice, in science as well as in art. In this regard we have to consider alcohol as the basis of other essences not less potent than itself.

The process of distillation of essences from liquids and from vegetable substances once established, it. was but natural that some adept should turn his hand to mineral bodies and try if they would not yield some new product that should be of effective and novel quality. Into the distillatory soon pass, therefore, all manner of things, from the horn of the stag or hart, to the skull and brain of the dead man. Among other substances there was submitted to distillation the green stony crystal found in the earth, and called green vitriol, in Latin *vitriolum.* The result of the distillation of this *vitriolum* was to obtain as a yield, in the retort, the heavy oily corrosive fluid called, originally, spirit of vitriol, called now oil of vitriol or sulphuric acid.

Many were the fanciful things thought of by the adepts concerning this oil, and even to the letters of which the word *vitriolum* is made up they attached a mystical symbolism. In course of time they began to combine and to distil other fluids with the corrosive sulphurous oil, and amongst the first of fluids used in this manner stood spirit of wine. The experiment did not deceive them, for it gave them as a product one of the most useful and wonderful of liquids. To them this new liquid as it first was taken from the retort was an infinite marvel. They poured it on water and it floated, on spirit and it floated. They poured it into their hands, and, lo! it boiled there. It escaped from them into an invisible state or air before they could well bottle it; it burned and exploded. It caused, when it passed off from the surface of the living body, an intense cold. It dissolved wax, oil, fat, gums, resins, balsams, and yet when it was set free it let them fall again. It was so light that a measure which would hold ten pounds weight of water would only hold seven pounds of this light intangible liquid. What name shall they apply to this substance, the lightest known? They designate it by a term indicating the lightest thing they can conceive: they compare it with the refined medium, with which the philosophers imagine the firmament to be filled, and they give it the same name. They call it *æther*.

Of what strange after-use this magical fluid has been to man we all know. It was introduced early into medicine, and was well studied last century by Dr. Ward, and by Mr. Turner, of Liverpool. In our own time, it has been discovered to have the power of suspending sensation and sensibility after being inhaled by the lungs, and by its means there has been re-introduced to the world that beneficent and long lost art of rendering the body insensible to pain during surgical operations.

More recently by a study of the application of ether for the production of intense cold, I myself introduced that local use of it for benumbing the body, called the ether spray.

The value of this secondary alcohol to man is indeed inestimable. You know how valuable it has been in photography as the volatile solvent of collodion, and in other various departments of the fine and useful arts it has rendered equally good service.

From the distillation of *vitriolum* our adepts soon passed to other solid substances. They distilled saltpetre, and so got the spirit of nitre, which we call now nitric acid; they distilled common salt in combination with oil of vitriol, and so got spirit of salts (marine acid), which we call hydrochloric acid. Again, with these new spirits they distilled spirits of wine to obtain new ethers, nitrous and marine. Then a chemist, the Count de Laura-gnais, distilled together acetic acid and spirit of wine, by which process he obtained acetous ether. Thus by these double actions, a numerous series of useful ethers has been obtained, it were too long for me to enumerate.

From the observation of the fermentation of wine we derive, in a certain sense, our first knowledge of gases. Van Helmont gave to the gas which comes from the fermenting of vegetable matter the name of *gas sylvestre*, and from this may be dated the origin of the study of these invisible forms of matter. Priestley made some of his early observations on the gas which escaped from fermenting malt in a brewery at Warrington, and was led step by step to the liberation of gases from mineral and earthy substances, and so to the discovery of oxygen. Upon that discovery, coupled with his method of collecting gases by displacement of water, and of trying their qualities, came the process of distilling and collecting a gas from coal, and thus coal gas.

After the discovery of the element known as chlorine, and of the compounds of that element with other elements, another new era was opened in the history of alcohol. By passing chlorine through alcohol, Liebig obtained that narcotic substance which we call chloral hydrate; and by treating alcohol with chloride of lime, the same great experimentalist produced for us chloroform, an agent which has rivalled ether in its service as a soother and saver of pain. A glance at the table— No. IV. of the Appendix—of anæsthetics or sleep producers will show by the names in italics those substances which come from alcohol. All that have proved of most use excepting one, nitrous oxide or laughing gas, have this common origin.

Had the time not been expended, I could have brought before you further illustration upon illustration of these secondary uses of alcohol to man; but I must stop, content in having recalled to your minds some of the more striking facts in the history of the curious and important agent which is now the subject of our studies.

LECTURE II.

THE ALCOHOL GROUP OF ORGANIC BODIES— ACTIONS OF DIFFERENT ALCOHOLS.

IF before a chemist of a hundred years ago you could have placed a specimen of spirit of wine or alcohol, and could have asked him of what it was composed, he would have told you that it was the element of water combined with elementary fire, to which elementary fire he would give the name of phlogiston, a name derived from a Greek word signifying to burn or inflame. He would tell you that all bodies that burned were phlogisticated, and that bodies that would not burn were dephlogisticated. The substance that was left behind was, he would probably add, the element with which the elementary fire had previously been combined. Were you to ask him whence he derived this knowledge, he would say, "from the greatest chemist who had ever lived before his time, George Ernest Stahl, Professor of Medicine, Anatomy, and Chemistry in the University of Halle, who had died in Berlin, whither he had gone to be physician to the King of Prussia, forty years ago."

As proof that alcohol was elementary water combined with phlogiston, our ancient chemist would probably show you this experiment:—He would place a portion of the spirit in a cup, would set fire to the spirit, and would invert over the flame a glass vessel, shaped almost like a common globe, which he would call a cucurbit, into which he would allow the flame to ascend. He would indicate that within the glass vessel a vapor, derived from the burning fluid, formed and condensed, as you see it forming and condensing now. Collecting this fluid, he would prove to you that it was water, which water he could show to be nothing else but one indivisible thing, therefore an element. Thus his demonstration would be complete. The element, while it existed as spirit, yielded fire on burning; it was fire water. The fire was condensed with the water. Nothing could be plainer, according to his light of science.

If you had inquired of the chemist whether he had any symbol by which to denote elementary water or spirit, he would give you, as a symbol for water, a sign something like the letter V, with two wavy lines following the letters; and for spirit of wine, a sign like the letter V with the letter S in the centre, as I put it on the blackboard; and if once more you questioned him as to whether his laboratory contained any similar chemical substance, he would answer—none. Spirit of wine stood by itself a pure substance, possessing single and special virtues.

If, passing over the intervening hundred years, you asked the chemist of to-day, "What is alcohol?" he would tell you that it was an organic radical called ethyl, combined with the elements of water. He would explain that water was no longer considered to be an element, but to be composed of two elements, called hydrogen and oxygen, two equivalents of hydrogen being combined in it with one equivalent of oxygen. He would inform you that the radical he had called ethyl was a compound of carbon and hydrogen, and he would add that this radical in alcohol took the place of one of the equivalents of hydrogen of water. He thereupon would give you symbols for water and alcohol, but symbols of a very different kind to those presented by his learned predecessor. He would express the names of the elements composing the water and spirit by the first letters of their names, and add their equivalents, or parts, by figures attached to the letters. Thus his symbol for water would be H_2O; for the radical ethyl, C_2H_5; and for alcohol $(C_2H_5) HO$ or C_2H_6O.

Were you interested about the theory of phlogiston, invented by the illustrious George Ernest Stahl, your modern guide would instruct you that the theory had long since been discarded, and that towards the latter part of the last century the very books of its discoverer had been burned, in derision, by a priestess of science in one of the temples of science in Paris. Then through what a wonderful history of discovery during the hundred years he would, if he liked, lead you. Into this cucurbit in which I burned the alcohol, and which you will observe I closed by placing it with its mouth downwards upon the table, he would pour clear lime water as I do now; he would shake the water round the sides of the cucurbit and see, as he did it, the water would become milky white.

This phenomenon he would indicate was due to the presence of a gas which the old chemist had actually collected but had overlooked. That gas is carbonic acid. It, as well as the water, was the product of the combustion of the spirit, and it now, in combination with the lime water, has united with the lime, forming carbonate of lime or chalk. Following the history of this gas, called once fixed air, because it could thus be fixed by lime and other substances, he would show how it had been proved to consist of carbon and oxygen; how it is given off from the burning of bodies containing carbon; and how a French chemist of the last century, named Lavoisier, traced out by analysis that, in fermentation, the juice of grapes is changed from being sweet and full of sugar into a vinous liquor, which no longer contains any sugar, the inflammable liquor known as spirit of wine. Thence it would be shown that the same illustrious chemist, making an analysis of sugar and studying the effects of yeast in causing fermentation of sugar, collected and weighed the elements produced, determined the elementary composition of spirit as consisting of carbon, hydrogen, and oxygen, and from his research announced the new principle in chemistry, that in all the operations in art and nature nothing is created; that an equal quantity of matter exists both before and after the experiment; that the quality and quantity of the elements remain precisely the same; that nothing takes place beyond changes and modifications in the combinations of the elements; and that in every chemical experiment an exact equality must

be supposed between the elements of the body examined, and those of the products of its analysis.
Finally, on this head, he would state the theory of
Lavoisier, that *must* consists of alcohol combined
with carbonic acid, and that the effects of vinous
fermentation upon sugar are reduced to the mere separation of the elements of sugar into two portions ;
one portion oxygenated at the expense of the other,
so as to form carbonic acid ; the other disoxyge-
nated to form alcohol; so that were it possible to
reunite alcohol and carbonic acid the product
would be sugar.　Bringing you down to a later
period, the modern chemist would describe a theory current about between thirty and forty years
ago that alcohol is a compound of olefiant gas and
water, and that in a state of vapor it consists of
equal volumes of these.　Or, again, that it was a
hydrate of ether; or, again, according to a still
later view, that it was a hydrated oxide of ethyl.
Thus he would bring you to the latest theory as
to composition which I have already supplied.

　Lastly, if for the sake of further comparison you
asked the chemist of to-day whether alcohol had
any ally or congener, he would reply, many.　He
would give you, for instance, this spirit, which he
would call methylic alcohol, and which he would
tell you was got also by distillation, only that the
distillation was dry, and that the substance distilled was wood ; or he would give you this specimen, which he would call amylic alcohol, and
which he would tell you was got by distillation,
not of wood, but of potato.　Again, he would show
you other specimens, to which he would give

different names as indicated in table No. V. of the Appendix.

Directing your attention to the composition of these alcohols, the chemist would beg you to observe that their chemical construction is throughout the same, that is to say, in all cases, a radical composed of carbon and hydrogen has replaced one of the equivalents of hydrogen of water. The radicals, however, vary in respect to the equivalents of the elements of which they are composed, and to distinguish them they have different names. Essentially each radical, though it is composed of more than one element, acts as if it were one, and is called a base, because it is a root or origin upon which other structures rest. Thus, in the present case, the radicals, as they vary in amount of carbon and hydrogen which they contain, produce, in each case of their combination with water, an alcohol possessing a different property or different properties from the other alcohols. The table No. VI. of the Appendix will give an illustration of the increase of carbon and hydrogen in the radicals of the series.

The first of the radicals, methyl, is composed of one equivalent of carbon and three of hydrogen. The radical ethyl of two of carbon and five of hydrogen. The radical propyl of three of carbon and seven of hydrogen, and so on, the increase in the equivalents of the elements being after a given rule in the whole series, the carbon increasing one, and the hydrogen two with each progressive step. So, as the alcohols progressively change from the first of the series, the methylic, they grow richer in carbon and hydrogen, and proportionately they grow heavier, less soluble, and less volatile.

A very simple experiment suffices to show the increase of carbon in these series. If I take a piece of cotton wool, place it in a glass cup, pour upon it a little methylic alcohol, in which alcohol there is the smallest amount of carbon, set fire to it and hold a white plate over the flame, the plate remains white because the air that reaches the flame is sufficient to consume all the carbon. If I do the same experiment with ethylic alcohol, although the carbon is a little greater, yet the result remains the same. If I move two steps higher, viz., to butylic alcohol, in which there are four equivalents of carbon, the combustion is not quite complete, and therefore a shade or stain of carbon is left on the plate : and if, going one step further in the series, I use amylic alcohol, then the combustion is rendered so imperfect that a thick layer of carbon, derived from the alcohol, in the destruction of it by the burning, is left upon the white surface. I may digress here for a moment to state,—if the practical fact about to be told be considered a digression,—that this simple mode of testing common alcohol will serve roughly to detect extreme adulteration of it with the heavier alcohol—fusel oil, some of which I last burnt. This heavier alcohol is used in adulteration, and as you will learn when you hear of its effects, it is a dangerous adulterant. I was dining a few months ago with some friends, one of whom produced a small flask of precious liquor he had had presented to him, and which was said to be an

unusually choice hollands. On examining it I felt
sure it was a gin treated with fusel oil, and on
burning a little of it, this suspicion was confirmed
by a deposit of carbon upon a white dish.   I
warned my friends forthwith of the danger of
drinking this heavy, though certainly pleasant
spirit, and the majority took the warning. Two,
less prudent, indulged, to suffer for the next two
or three succeeding days to an extent that con-
vinced them that there was no mistake in the
scientific and friendly admonition they had received.

The physical distinctions between the various
alcohols now before us are marked by other signs.
For example, as we move from the methylic alcohol upwards, we discover that their vapors increase in weight, that as fluids they grow heavier,
and that their boiling point, that is to say the temperature required to make them boil, has to be
increased.   Another table, No. VII. of the Appendix, illustrates these facts in relation to four alcohols of the series : viz., methylic, ethylic, butylic,
and amylic.

Thus the vapor density of methylic alcohol is 16
when compared with hydrogen gas as a standard ;
of ethylic alcohol, 23 ; of butylic, 37 ; and of amylic, 44.   In respect to the specific gravity of the
fluids, that is to say of the weights of the fluids
themselves, compared with water estimated as a
thousand, the same rule extends, with the one
remarkable exception, viz., that the methylic alcohol appears heavier than the ethylic, after which
the weights increase, so that amylic alcohol stands

as 811, to 792 the weight of ethylic. Again, as to the boiling points, the lightest alcohol boils at 140, that is 72° below the boiling point of water; ethylic at 172; propylic at 205; butylic at 230, or 18° above the boiling point of water; and amylic at 270, or 58° above the boiling point of water, on Fahrenheit's scale.

The analogies between these various alcohols are sustained throughout by other chemical changes relating to them. If we expose diluted common alcohol to the atmosphere under fitting conditions it becomes acidified; in other words, it is converted into vinegar. This is due to its oxydation, in which process there are two steps; one by which the spirit is converted into a substance called aldehyde (dehydrated alcohol—al-de-hyd), and then into acetic acid, or vinegar. In the formation of the aldehyde two atoms of the hydrogen are oxydised, by which water is produced, and the aldehyde has therefore the composition of C_2H_4O. In the formation of the acetic acid another atom of oxygen is added, and the acetic acid has therefore the composition of $C_2H_4O_2$. This same series of changes extends through all the alcohols, as will be seen from table No. VIII. of the Appendix.

I said, in the first lecture, that from common or ethylic alcohol a new compound can be obtained by heating it with sulphuric acid, to which compound the name of ether is applied. In like manner, an ether can be obtained from the other alcohols.

If chlorine be brought to bear upon ethylic

alcohol, the elements of water, that is to say, the oxygen and the hydrogen are removed, and are replaced by chlorine, and there is formed chloride of ethyl. This change can be extended to all the other alcohols, the properties of the products being modified by the base.

The same rule extends to the action of iodine, and to that of nitrous acid. Tables IX. to XII. of the Appendix afford illustrations of these facts. They could be largely extended, but they are sufficient for our purpose.

I have brought for those who are curious to see them, twelve specimens of the different compounds formed on the alcohols. Six of these belong to the ethyl, or common alcohol series, six to the amyl, and they include respectively specimens of the alcohols, of the acids of the alcohols, of the ethers, of the chlorides, of the iodides, and of the nitrites. One of these specimens, I mean the nitrite of amyl, has within these last few years obtained a remarkable importance owing to its extraordinary action upon the body. A distinguished chemist, Professor Guthrie, while distilling over nitrite of amyl from amylic alcohol, observed that the vapor, when inhaled, quickened his circulation, and made him feel as if he had been running. There was flushing of his face, rapid action of his heart, and breathlessness. In 1861–2, I made a careful and prolonged study of the action of this singular body, and discovered that it produced its effect by causing an extreme relaxation, first, of the blood vessels, and afterwards of the muscular fibres of the body. To such an extent did this agent relax, I found it would even overcome the tetanic spasm produced by strychnia, and having thus discovered its action, I ventured to propose its use for removing the spasm in some of the extremest spasmodic diseases. The results have more than realised my expectations. Under the influence of this agent, one of the most agonising of known human maladies, called *Angina pectoris*, has been brought under such control that the paroxysms have been regularly prevented, and in one instance, at least, altogether removed. Even tetanus, or lock-jaw has been subdued by it, and in two instances, of an extreme kind so effectively as to warrant the credit of what may be truly called a cure. I notice this action of nitrite of amyl because it will be referred to again in explanation of certain of the effects of alcohol.

I should have liked, if there had been time, to have dwelt at greater length on many other interesting points bearing on these different alcohols and their derivatives. I should have been pleased to have presented to you a more extended account of the progress of discovery during the past century leading to these modern facts; and I should much have liked to have rendered more complete the description of the alcohol series of bodies, by explaining the differences of what are called monatomic, diatomic, and triatomic alcohols; but I must desist for two reasons; first, because the study would lead me into too great detail, and secondly, because it would introduce to notice a series of compounds, the physiological action of which are not so well understood as are those to which I shall soon direct your attention and the study of which is more than enough for the time that is at our disposal. It must be considered sufficient, therefore, if I have succeeded in showing that the common alcohol is but one of a group of a series of chemical compounds, and that its superior claim to our notice rests upon its antiquity as a discovered substance, and on its enormous distribution in civilised communities, rather than on its special or distinctive properties as a chemical agent.

One other series of facts I would, however, briefly describe before leaving this part of my subject. If into this ethylic alcohol I throw a portion of the metal sodium, a brisk action immediately begins to take place; as you will see, a gas escapes which I easily collect in a glass tube, which burns, and if mixed with air, explodes, as you hear. The gas is hydrogen. A change of substitution has occurred in this experiment. The hydrogen belonging to the water of the alcohol has been replaced by the sodium, and what is called sodium alcohol is produced. The result would have been the same with potassium as the replacing metal.

By acting on common alcohol with strong potash, then with sulphuretted hydrogen, and afterwards with iodide of ethyl, a new alcohol is produced called mercaptan. In this fluid the oxygen of the alcohol is replaced by sulphur, so that the formula for it is (C_2H_5) HS. It is a fluid, whitish in color, and of so offensive and penetrating an odor that it can hardly be approached until it is largely diluted with common alcohol. It is nearly insoluble in water, but imparts to it its peculiar odor; its specific gravity is 832, compared with water as 1,000; it is thirty-one times heavier than hydrogen, and it boils at 135° Fahr.

Sulphur alcohol is very rarely seen, but there is a diluted specimen here which has been prepared with very great care. There is only 5 per cent. of it in the solution, and yet its odor is as strong as can well be borne.

From this point I proceed to dwell on the action of certain of the alcohols which have been brought before us up to the present time, excluding on this occasion the alcohol best known, I mean the common alcohol of commerce, or as we know it chemically, ethylic alcohol. The point I shall aim at will be to show the influence of these alcohols upon animal life, and thereby to lead up to the action of ethylic alcohol pure and simple. The subject is one entirely new, and is limited to a very few bodies of the alcohol group, viz., to methylic alcohol, butylic, amylic, the potassium and sodium alcohols, and sulphur alcohol or mercaptan.

ACTION OF METHYLIC ALCOHOL.

Methylic alcohol, pyroxylic spirit or wood spirit, as it has been differently called, the spirit contained in the liquid got by distilling wood, has been known for about 62 years. It was discovered by Mr. Philip Taylor, in 1812, and was soon applied for lamps and for other purposes as a spirit. It was prob-

ably first made commercially by Messrs. Turnbull
and Ramsay, of Glasgow. Its properties were in-
vestigated and reported upon by Sir Robert Kane,
of Dublin, in 1836, and it was also analysed by
Messrs. Dumas and Peligot, who determined that
it contained 37.5 per cent. of carbon, 12.5 per cent.
of hydrogen, and 50 per cent. of oxygen. When it
is pure it remains clear in the atmosphere. It has
an aromatic smell, with a slight acidity. The
specimen I have used for my research had a specific weight of 810, water being 1,000, and it boiled
at 140° Fahr.

The spirit has been much used in the arts in the
place of alcohol for making varnishes. Having a
lower boiling point it is more volatile than common alcohol. It is now also largely used in museums for preserving purposes, and it yields on
oxydation a very powerful preservative vinegar.
For the sake of economy it is often employed in
the manufacture of other compounds called methy-
lated.

Owing to the volatile nature of this alcohol it
may be exhibited freely by inhalation in the same
manner that chloroform is administered. It then
enters the blood by being carried with the air that
is inspired into the pulmonary tract, and thus into
the air vesicles. Here it is absorbed into the circulation by the minute blood-vessels which make
their way from the heart over the lungs, and which
ramify upon the vesicles. By administrating th·
vapor of methylic alcohol in this way its effects
are rapidly developed, for it condenses quickly in
the blood, is carried rapidly into the left side of

the heart, and thence is distributed by the arteries over the whole body as quickly as it is condensed and absorbed.

The alcohol may be administered in the usual way, that is to say, in combination with water, hot or cold. In this way it is not unpleasant to the taste, and in one instance, as I am informed by a veteran member of my profession, this alcohol was invariably drunk by a well-known physician, in preference to common alcohol. He was accustomed to make it into toddy, with water and sugar, and considered that while it was as pleasant to take as ordinary spirituous drinks, it was less injurious than they are. I have myself, of late years, when compelled to allow the administration of alcohol, sometimes recommended this methylic lighter spirit, and I am satisfied, with better results than if the heavier or ethylic spirit had been employed. I have ventured also to suggest that in many instances other physicians might follow the same practice with advantage ; for methylic alcohol is much more rapid in its action, and much less prolonged in its effects than is common alcohol, so that it produces its effects promptly, and what is of most importance, it demands the least possible ultimate expenditure of animal force for its elimination from the body. This latter fact, I repeat, is of great moment, for, in the end, all these alcoholic fluids are depressants, and although at first, by their calling vigorously into play the natural forces, they seem to excite and are therefore called stimulants, they themselves supply no force at any time, but cause expenditure of force, by which means they get away out of the body and therewith lead to exhaustion and paralysis of motion. In other words, the animal force which should be expended on the nutrition and sensation of the body, is in part expended on the alcohol, an entirely foreign expenditure.

The lighter the alcohol therefore, *cæteris paribus*, the less injurious its action, and so we may put down methylic alcohol as the safest of the series of bodies to which it belongs. But it is not without potency of effect, and the phenomena it produces are sufficiently demonstrative. Its effects are developed in four distinct stages.

The first stage is that of excitement of the nervous organisation; the pulse is quickened, the breathing is quickened, the surface of the body is flushed, and the pupil is dilated. After a little time there is a sense of languor, the muscles falling into a state of prostration and the muscular movements becoming irregular. Thereupon the second stage follows, if the administration be continued. In this second stage the muscular prostration is increased, the breathing is labored, and is attended by deep sighing movements at intervals of about four or five seconds, followed by further prostration, rolling over of the body upon the side, and distinct signs of intoxication. From this condition the subject passes into the third stage, which is that of entire intoxication, complete insensibility to pain, with unconsciousness of all external objects, and with inability to exert any voluntary muscular power. The breathing now becomes embarrassed and blowing, with what is techni-

cally called "bronchial rale," or rattle, due to the
passage of air through fluid that has accumulated
in the finer bronchial passages. The heart and
lungs, however, even in this stage, retain their
functions, and therefore recovery will take place
if the conditions for it be favorable. Also, if the
body be touched or irritated in parts, there will
be response of motion, not from any knowledge or
consciousness, but from what we physiologists call
"reflex action;" that is to say, the impression we
have made by irritation upon the surface of the
body has travelled by its usual route through the
nerves to its nervous centre in the brain, and uncontrolled there by the consciousness has rolled
back again, stimulating in its course some muscular fibre to motion. Probably the reason why the
heart, which is a muscle, and the breathing muscles, continue to beat while all the other portions
are at rest is due to this fact, that the blood which
the heart drives to the brain and other nervous
centres conveys to the centres which supply the
heart a wave of motion that rolls back upon these
vital muscles, and sustains them still in their
rhythmical motion.

During all these stages there is no violent convulsive action from this alcohol, and no distinct
tremor; but one phenomenon has been step by
step more marked, and that phenomenon is a reduction of the animal temperature. Even though
the body of the subject be exposed to a temperature of 84°, that is summer heat, it will begin to
cool from the first, and will continue to cool
through all the stages, so that at last the loss of

heat will become actually dangerous; for the cold body cannot throw off water freely, and therefore fluid collects in the lungs, and there is risk of what may be plainly considered suffocation like as from drowning. I have seen this decline of temperature from methylic alcohol, in animals narcotised by it, proceed to the loss of eight degrees of heat on Fahrenheit's scale when the insensibility was at its extreme point.

Presuming that the administration of the methylic spirit be continued when the third degree has been reached, there is a last stage, which is that of death. The two remaining nervous centres which feed the heart and respiration cease simultaneously to act, and all motion is over. After the death the blood throughout the body is found charged with the alcohol. The circulation of blood over the lungs has continued to the last, and so the lungs are found containing blood in both sides of the heart; the vessels of the brain are engorged with blood, as are the other vascular organs. The blood itself is not materially changed in physical quality, but coagulates, or forms into clot, rather more slowly than usual.

If at the third stage of insensibility the administration of methylic spirit be stopped, recovery from the insensibility and prostration will invariably take place on one condition, that the body be kept dry and warm. From four to five hours, however, are necessary before the recovery is complete, and under the best conditions the restoration of the animal temperature is not perfected under a period of seven hours.

Happily we have no data to guide us that will show the effects on the animal body of the long continued use of methylic alcohol, for men have not as yet so steadily plied themselves with it as a drink as to induce phenomena of chronic intoxication from it. The above-named facts, however, drawn from careful observations, in which the effects of the agent were seen on the inferior animals, and in one instance where the fluid was taken by accident by the human subject, show that methylic alcohol, though it may be less potent than its allies, is sufficiently potent, and the inference is fair, indeed irresistible, that if the use of it were persevered in for long periods of time, it would lead to structural change in the body, just as all other chemical agents do that modify and pervert the natural mechanism. An agent that causes congestion of the brain cannot be employed many times without destroying the delicate organisation of the vascular structure of the brain, neither can it influence the other vascular organs in the same way without prejudice to their structure; neither can it destroy the function of the nerves, of the muscles, and of the organs of the senses without prejudice to their functions. In many respects this, the lightest and least injurious of the alcohols, resembles chloroform in the ultimate action it produces on the body. It still more closely resembles ether, although recovery from the effects of both these agents is very much more rapid than from the spirit. It may consequently, as a chemical agent possessing a specific power of action over the living organism, be fairly classified with

these agents. It is quite as artificial as they are,
it is quite as dangerous in the long run, and its
effects are more prolonged.

ACTION OF BUTYLIC ALCOHOL.

I pass over the second alcohol of our series, viz.,
ethylic alcohol, the common alcohol of wines and
spirits, because that will of itself engage our attention for the remaining part of the course, after this
lecture is concluded. I pass over propylic also for
the reason that it is not easily separated as an
alcohol, and is less perfectly studied than the other
members of the group before us. Thus I am
brought to what is called butylic alcohol.

With this spirit we arrive at one of the heavier
bodies of the group in which, as our table shows,
there is a higher proportion of carbon and hydrogen than exists in those that are placed above it in
the scale. Compared with common alcohol the
weight of its vapor is as 37 to 23. Its weight, as a
fluid, is 803 to 792, and its boiling point 230 Fahr.
to 172. It is a heavier fluid ; it mixes indifferently
with water, but it is not unpleasant to take when
diluted and sweetened. Applied to the lips and
tongue when in a pure state it creates a sensation
of burning, in the same way as common spirit, but
with more intensity, and there is this remarkable
fact connected with the sensation, that after the
burning effect has passed away an extreme numb-
ness of the part, where the fluid was applied, remains. I made this observation originally in 1869,
and I have since often applied the knowledge with

effect, in relieving, by the application of the agent,
local pain. Toothache, for instance, is very quickly
soothed by it.

The alcohol is not obtained by a special process
of distillation ; it is produced with other alcohols
in the process of fermentation, and is obtained by
what is called fractional distillation, that is, by distillation of it, at certain fixed temperatures, from
fusel oil, or from the oil of beet-root, or from mo-
lasses after distillation of ethylic spirit.

The action of butylic alcohol on the animal body
is divisible into four stages, the same as we have
seen in respect to methylic spirit, but the period
required for producing the different stages is
greatly prolonged ; and when the third stage, that
of complete insensibility, is reached, there is added
a new phenomenon which does not belong to any
of the lighter alcohols. In this third degree, after
the temperature of the body is depressed to the
minimum by the butylic spirit, distinct tremors
occur throughout the whole of the muscular system. These come on at regular intervals spontaneously, but they can be excited by a touch at
any time, and in the intervals where they are
absent there is frequent twitching of the muscles.
The tremors themselves are not positively muscular contractions, but are rather vibrations or wave-
like motions through the muscles, and are attended
with an extreme deficiency of true contractile
power in the muscular fibre. An electrical current passed through the muscles, which would, in
health, throw them into rigid contraction, will
now excite the tremors and keep them proceeding,

but will not excite complete contraction. So long as the tremors are present, the temperature of the body is depressed, falling even half a degree ; but when they cease the temperature rises again, not to the natural standard, but to or near that which existed before the tremors were excited. After the tremors are once established, they continue without further administration of the alcohol for ten and twelve hours, and so slowly do they decline, they may remain in a slight degree for even thirty-six hours. They subside by remission of intensity and prolongation of interval of recurrence. One fact of singular significance attaches itself to these muscular tremors. They are the tremors which occur in man during the stage of alcoholic disease, when there is set up that malady to which we give the name of *delirium tremens.* An ordinary intoxication with a lighter alcohol is insufficient to produce this extreme perversion of nervous and muscular power, but the introduction of one of these heavier alcohols, or, it may be, the excessive saturation of the body with a lighter spirit, for on this point I am not sure, is sufficient to cause the tremulous motion. What the nature of these muscular movements is, what unnatural relationships exist between the nervous system, the muscles, and the blood, to lead to them are questions still unsolved. Involuntary, developed even against the will, excited by any external touch, attended with great reduction of temperature, and remaining as long as the temperature is reduced, they indicate an extreme depression of animal force : a condition in which all the force of

life that remains has to be expended on the more
organic acts of life, on the support of the motions
of the heart, the muscles of respiration, and the
functions of the secreting glands. The voluntary
systems of nerve and muscle are indeed well-nigh
dead, and recovery rests entirely on the maintenance of the organic nervous power. Still recovery
will take place if the body be sustained by external
heat and by internal nourishment.

In the extreme stage of intoxication from butylic
alcohol the red blood in the arteries loses its rich
color, and the blood from the veins, which flows
with difficulty, is of a dirty hue. The blood
coagulates readily, but the clot is loose, and the
fibrine of which it is composed separates in a
coarse network or mesh. The little corpuscles of
the blood run into each other, forming rolls or
columns. Indeed, it is wonderful how the blood
circulates through the structures it should nourish.
The vascular membranes of the brain are found
charged with this tarry blood; the brain structure
is softened, and gives the odor of the poison, and
the muscles, when divided by the knife, cut without firmness, yielding from numerous points the
same tar-like blood. The vascular organs—spleen,
liver, lungs, kidneys—are equally changed, and in
a similar manner. Their fine structures are infil-
trated with the deteriorated vascular fluid which
was intended for their maintenance, and even the
secretions and cavities of the body are perverted
by being charged with fluid derived from the unnatural blood. This is the state of the body of one
who dies insensible after the delirium and tremors

which characterise the human malady, self-inflicted and terrible, known as *delirium tremens.*

ACTION OF AMYLIC ALCOHOL.

Amylic alcohol, the next of our series, is obtained by the fermentation of potato starch, or starch of grain, and when pure is a colorless fluid. Its weight, compared with water as 1,000, is 818, and it boils at 270° Fahr. It is from this alcohol that the active substance, nitrite of amyl, to which I have before referred, is derived. The odor of amylic alcohol is sweet, nauseous, and heavy. The sensation of its presence remains long. In taste it is burning and acrid, and it is itself practically insoluble in water. When it is diluted with common alcohol it dissolves freely in water, and gives a soft and rather unctuous flavor, I may call it a fruity flavor, something like that of ripe pears. From the quantities of it imported into this country it is believed to be employed largely in the adulteration of wines and spirits.

Amylic alcohol, when it is introduced as an adulterant, is an extremely dangerous addition to ordinary alcohol, in whatever form it is presented, whether as wine or spirit. Its action on the body is the same as that of butylic alcohol. It produces three stages of insensibility, ending in the profoundest narcotism, or coma, followed by reduction of temperature and by muscular tremors. These tremors recur with the most perfect regularity of themselves, but they can be excited at any moment by touching the body, or blowing upon it, or even by a sharp noise, such as the snap of the finger. In all other respects the phenomena induced are the same as are observed from butylic alcohol, except that they are much more prolonged, from two to three days being sometimes required for the complete restoration of the animal temperature. The reason of this prolongation of action lies in the greater weight and the greater insolubility of this spirit ; that is to say, the force required to decompose it, or mechanically to lift it out of the body when it has once entered it, is so much greater than is required for the lighter spirits, which diffuse more readily through the secretions, volatilise by the breath or possibly undergo rapid decomposition. The odor of the substance remains for many hours in the animal tissues. Amylic alcohol acts upon some resins and resinous substances, dissolving, I believe, certain of them more easily than the lighter spirits, but its peculiar odor prevents its application on a large scale.

ACTION OF SODIUM AND POTASSIUM ALCOHOLS.

The action of the sodium and potassium alcohols is exceedingly interesting in a physiological, although not in a practical point of view, except in respect to their various uses as chemical re-agents. They act on the living animal tissues as caustics, and will one day be considered of great service to the surgeon. Brought into contact with blood, in solution, there is produced by them an almost instant crystallisation of needle-like crystals spread out in beautiful arborescent filaments. This arborescent appearance is identical with a crystallisation which can be induced in these alcohors themselves, but there are also formed smaller radiant crystals due to the crystallisation of the crystalloidal matter of the blood-cells, and singularly like the forms which, since the time of Dr. Richard Mead, have been described as occurring in the blood after infection by the poison of the viper.

These metallic alcohols are powerful antiseptics, like common alcohol, over which they have an advantage in that they more thoroughly harden soft structures. I have taken advantage of this action to employ them for the preservation of nervous matter, which is rapidly prone to decomposition.

I should add that, by some chemists these alcohols are called ethylates of sodium or potassium, a term which is thought to define more correctly their chemical construction.

ACTION OF MERCAPTAN OR SULPHUR ALCOHOL.

I have already referred briefly to this most curious body of the alcohol series, describing it as an alcohol in which oxygen is replaced by sulphur. In experimenting with it a solution containing 5 per cent. is sufficient, and the vapor of it may be inhaled in order to produce its effects. These are most remarkable.

I found, by direct experiment, that the vapor is not irritating to breathe, but that its influence on the system is speedily pronounced. There is a desire for sleep, and a strange, unhappy sensation, as if some actual or impending trouble were at hand. This is succeeded by an easy but extreme sensation of muscular fatigue; the limbs feel too heavy to be lifted, and rest is absolutely necessary. There is, at the same time, no insensibility to pain, and no intoxication. The pulse is rendered feeble and slow, and remains so for one or two hours; but, in time, all the effects pass off, and active motion in the air helps quickly to dispose of them.

On the inferior animals the action of mercaptan is equally peculiar. Frogs exposed to its vapor fall asleep, and seem to pass into actual death, except that the eye remains bright. They may be left in this apparently lifeless state for half an hour, then, removed into the air, they commence, in the course of an hour and a half or two hours, to breathe again, and gradually recover, precisely as if they were awaking from sleep. The action of this alcohol on the animal body, though it produces these extreme effects, is less injurious than that of the other alcohols. It escapes rapidly by the breath, and in some new form, as a sulphur compound. It communicates to the breath an odor which is by no means uncommon in persons who indulge to a great extent in the use of ordinary alcohol. This observation suggests a most important explanation of certain phenomena connected with the action of common alcohol. It appears to me that in some states there is actually produced in the living organism, by the vital chemistry, sulphur compounds, derived probably from the bile, a substance rich in sulphur, which

compounds, distributed by the blood to the nervous matter, create phenomena similar to those I
have described as following upon the inhalation of
mercaptan. Thus, under unnatural modes of life,
the body may actually make its own poisons, and
the doctor be often asked to remove what the
patient, if he were a better chemist and a wiser
man, would never produce for the exercise of the
doctor's skill.

LECTURE III.

THE primary action of ethylic alcohol on animal
life forms our next study. This is the alcoholic
spirit which enters into wines, beers, and ordinary
spirituous liquors.

There are two modes in which this subject must
be discussed. One relates to the mere physical
action of alcohol upon the body, the other to its
action as a food for the body. Of the varied substances which we take into our systems, some, like
chloroform, or opium, produce very marked physical effects, which we may call physiological, but
which have nothing to do with the nourishment of
the organism, nor with the sustainment of its vital
power. Other substances act as foods, producing
certain continuous phenomena of structural build
and of vital function. Alcohol is peculiar in that
we are obliged to consider it, at the present time,
from each of these points of view, and I now take
up the first, I mean the purely physical action of
alcohol, reserving the question of its qualities as a
food for a future lecture.

A very simple problem lies before us. The sum
of £117,000,000 of money is invested in this country
on alcohol as a commercial substance. Where

does the alcohol go? We know that the larger part of it goes for consumption by human beings. A little—I mean, by comparison, a little—is used for the purposes of art and science, but the greater portion of it, practically all but the whole of it, is consumed by human beings. Thus a question arises, we may almost say, of engineering and commerce, a question, therefore, particularly worthy of this Society, viz., What is the good of this invested capital, and of the substance which it supplies? It is not necessary for any of us to consider ourselves as physicians in studying this matter, but we may all consider ourselves as animal engineers, anxious to know the physical properties of agents which influence the animal life. To put it in a very practical way, suppose that there was no question involved in regard to the influence of alcohol upon the body, but that in the course of the invention of motive engines—common inanimate engines, which can be made to exhibit motive power by the application of heat to water—it had originally become the practice from some circumstance to put into the engines so much spirit with the water, and to work the engines with this mixture. Then suppose somebody said, " This is a very expensive process of working the engines ; may be they will work as well without the spirit." You would naturally inquire, " Can such be fact ? " And you would seek an engineer to fill the place I have now the honor to occupy, to explain to you the mechanism of the engines. You would also beg him to explain and put before you facts which would bear upon the point, whether the admixture of spirit and water was useful or useless? Now, please, consider me to-night as an engineer, and the animal body as the engine I am to speak upon. I am not going to address a word to you as a physician; I am not going to offer advice. I simply mean to place before you, as far as I know them, the facts relating to the physical effects of this thing, alcohol, when it is put into one of those millions of engines which we call men.

Alcohol will enter the body—the engine of which I am about to speak—by many channels. It can be introduced by injecting it under the skin or into a vein. Exalted by heat into the form of vapor, it may be inhaled by man or animal, when it will penetrate into the lungs, will diffuse through the bronchial tubes, will pass into the minute air vesicles of the lungs, will travel through the minute circulation with the blood that is going over the air vesicles to the heart, will condense in that blood, will go direct to the left side of the heart, thence into the arterial canals and so throughout the body. Or, again, the spirit can be taken in by the more ordinary channel, the stomach. Through this channel it finds its way, by two routes, into the circulation. A certain portion of it—the greater portion of it—is absorbed direct by the veins of the alimentary surface, finds its way straight into the larger veins, which lead up to the heart, and onwards with the course of the blood. Another portion is picked up by those small structures which proceed from below the mucous surface of the stomach, which are called *villi*, and from which originate a series of fine tubes that reach at last the lower portion of a common tube known as the thoracic duct, the tube which ascends in front of the spinal column, and terminates at the junction of two large veins on the left side of the body, at a point where the venous blood, returning from the left arm, joins with the returning blood from the left side of the head on its way to the heart.

Thus in whatever way the alcohol is introduced it enters the blood; the shortest way is that by inhalation, the longest and most ordinary way is by the stomach. Indeed, except for experimental purposes, the introduction is always by this latter and longest route, and we may, for our practical purposes, only think of alcohol as a fluid taken by the mouth into the stomach, and absorbed like a food or a drink from the surface of the alimentary canal.

Suppose, then, a certain measure of alcohol be taken into the stomach, it will be absorbed there, but, previous to absorption, it will have to undergo a proper degree of dilution with water, for there is this peculiarity respecting alcohol when it is separated by an animal membrane from a watery fluid like the blood, that it will not pass through the membrane until it has become charged, to a given point of dilution, with water. It is itself, in fact, so greedy for water, it will pick it up from watery textures, and deprive them of it until, by its saturation, its power of reception is exhausted, after which it will diffuse into the current of circulating fluid.

To illustrate this fact of dilution, I perform a simple experiment. Into a bladder is placed a mixture consisting of equal parts of alcohol and distilled water. Into the neck of the bladder a long glass tube is inserted and firmly tied. Then the bladder is immersed in a saline fluid representing an artificial serum of blood. The result is, that the alcohol in the bladder absorbs water from the surrounding saline solution, and thereby a column of fluid passes up into the glass tube. A second mixture of alcohol and water, in the proportion this time of one part of alcohol to two of water, is put into another bladder immersed in like manner in an artificial serum. In this instance, a little fluid also passes from the outside into the bladder, so that there is a rise of water in the tube, but less than in the previous instance. A third mixture, consisting of one part of alcohol with three parts of water, is placed in another little bladder, and is also suspended in the artificial serum. In this case there is, for a time, a small rise of fluid in the tube connected with the bladder; but after a while, owing to the dilution which took place, a current from within outwards sets in, and the tube becomes empty. Thus each bladder charged originally with the same quantity of fluid contains at last a different quantity. The first contains more than it did originally; the second a little more; the third a little less. From the third absorption takes place, and if I keep changing and replacing the outer fluid which surrounds the bladder with fresh serum, I can in time, owing to the double current of water into the bladder through its coats, and of water and alcohol out of the bladder into the serum, remove all the alcohol.

In this way it is removed from the stomach into the circulating blood after it has been swallowed. When we dilute alcohol with water before drinking it we quicken its absorption. If we do not dilute it sufficiently it is diluted in the stomach by trans- udation of water in the stomach until the required reduction for its absorption; the current then sets in towards the blood, and passes into the circulat- ing canals by the veins.

All the returning veins end in the large trunks which terminate in the central organ of the circu- lation—the heart. The heart, a moving muscular organ, has four cavities; two above called the au- ricles, two below called the ventricles. The cavi- ties on the right side are called respectively the right auricle and right ventricle; the cavities on the left side are called respectively the left auricle and the left ventricle. The right auricle receives all the venous blood of the body, and transmits it to the right ventricle; the right ventricle drives the blood over the lungs where the blood is ar- terialised; the left auricle receives the blood from the lungs, and transmits it to the left ventricle, which in turn drives it through the arterial tubes over the whole of the body, whence it returns again by the veins to the right side of the heart, and so on, in continuous circuit.

Alcohol, therefore, entering the veins, makes its way in the course I have described through the right heart, through the lungs, through the left heart, through the body at large by the arteries. This is the course of its travel in the organism. What does it do as it makes the round?

As it passes through the circulation of the lungs it is exposed to the air, and some little of it, raised into vapor by the natural heat, is thrown off in expiration. If the quantity of it be large this loss may be considerable, and the odor of the spirit may be detected in the expired breath. If the quantity be small the loss will be comparatively little, as the spirit will be held in solution by the water in the blood. After it has passed through the lungs, and has been driven by the left heart over the arterial circuit, it passes into what is called the minute circulation, or the structural circulation of the organism. The arteries here extend into very small vessels, which are called arterioles, and from these infinitely small vessels spring the equally minute radicals or roots of the veins which are ultimately to become the great rivers bearing the blood back to the heart. In its passage through this minute circulation the alcohol finds its way to every organ. To this brain, to these muscles, to these secreting or excreting organs, nay even into this bony structure itself, it moves with the blood. In some of these parts which are not excreting, it remains for a time diffused, and in those parts where there is a large percentage of water it remains longer than in other parts. From some organs which have an open tube for conveying fluids away, as the liver and kidneys, it is thrown out or eliminated, and in this way a portion of it is ultimately removed from the body. The rest passing round and round with the circulation, is probably decomposed and carried off in new forms of matter; but concerning this, more on a future occasion.

When we know the course which the alcohol takes in its passage through the body, from the period of its absorption to that of its elimination, we are the better able to judge what physical changes it induces in the different organs and structures with which it comes in contact. It first reaches the blood, but, as a rule, the quantity of it that enters is insufficient to produce any material effect on that fluid. If, however, the dose taken be poisonous or semi-poisonous, then even the blood, rich as it is in water—and it contains seven hundred and ninety parts in a thousand—is affected. The alcohol is diffused through this water, and there it comes in contact with the other constituent parts, with the fibrine, that plastic substance which, when blood is drawn, clots and coagulates, and which is present in the proportion of from two to three parts in a thousand; with the albumen which exists in the proportion of seventy parts; with the salts which yield about ten parts; with the fatty matters; and lastly, with those minute, round bodies which float in myriads in the blood (which were discovered by the Dutch philosopher, Leuwenhock, as one of the first results of microscopical observation, about the middle of the seventeenth century), and which are called the blood globules or corpuscles. These last named bodies are, in fact, cells; their discs, when natural, have a smooth outline, they are depressed in the centre, and they are red in color; the color of the blood being derived from them. We have discovered in recent years that there exist other corpuscles or cells in the blood in much smaller quantity, which

are called white cells, and these different cells float
in the blood-stream within the vessels. The red
take the centre of the stream; the white lie ex-
ternally near the sides of the vessels, moving less
quickly. Our business is mainly with the red
corpuscles. They perform the most important
functions in the economy; they absorb, in great
part, the oxygen which we inhale in breathing, and
carry it to the extreme tissues of the body; they
absorb, in great part, the carbonic acid gas which
is produced in the combustion of the body in the
extreme tissues, and bring that gas back to the
lungs to be exchanged for oxygen there; in short,
they are the vital instruments of the circulation.

With all these parts of the blood, with the water,
fibrine, albumen, salts, fatty matter, and corpuscles,
the alcohol comes in contact when it enters the
blood, and, if it be in sufficient quantity, it produces disturbing action. I have watched this disturbance very carefully on the blood corpuscles,
for in some animals we can see these floating along
during life, and we can also observe them from
men who are under alcohol by removing a speck
of blood, and examining it with the microscope.
The action of the alcohol, when it is observable, is
varied. It may cause the corpuscles to run too
closely together, and to adhere in rolls; it may
modify their outline, making the clear-defined
smooth outer edge irregular or crenate, or even
starlike; it may change the round corpuscle into
the oval form, or, in very extreme cases it may
produce what I may call a truncated form of corpuscles, in which the change is so great that if we

did not trace it through all its stages we should be puzzled to know whether the object looked at were indeed a blood-cell. All these changes are due to the action of the spirit upon the water contained in the corpuscles; upon the capacity of the spirit to extract water from them. During every stage of modification of corpuscle thus described, their function to absorb and fix gases is impaired, and when the aggregation of the cells, in masses, is great, other difficulties arise, for the cells united together pass less easily than they should through the minute vessels of the lungs and of the general circulation, and impede the current, by which local injury is produced.

A further action upon the blood instituted by alcohol in excess, is upon the fibrine or the plastic colloidal matter. On this the spirit may act in two different ways, according to the degree in which it affects the water that holds the fibrine in solution. It may fix the water with the fibrine, and thus destroy the power of coagulation; or it may extract the water so determinately as to produce coagulation. These facts bear on a new and refined subject of research with which I must not trouble you further, except to add that the inquiry explains why in acute cases of poisoning by alcohol the blood is sometimes found quite fluid, at other times firmly coagulated in the vessels.

These are the only points I have time to touch upon in respect to the physical action of alcohol upon blood. I must pass next to blood vessels, and trace out the action upon those fine ramifications of the larger vessels which we call the minute circulation. Upon these parts the spirit exerts a singular influence, from which arise a series of phenomena, characteristic of action when even a moderate quantity of spirit is taken into the body. That we may follow out this position clearly, it is essential that I should for a few minutes put alcohol out of sight altogether and describe the mechanism and governance of this minute circulating system.

If any of you ever visited the Royal College of Physicians you would find there a system of blood-vessels dissected and traced out by the immortal discoverer of the circulation of the blood himself, William Harvey; and I think it would strike you, as you looked on, that all the organs of the body, which constitute the body in its entirety, are built upon these minute vessels. It is as though Harvey had suggested the thought that the vascular system was the primary part of the animal organisation, and that upon it were planted and developed all the structures. The arteries are all beautifully shown branching out into their extreme divisions and giving the outline of the limbs, of the brain, of the visceral parts, and of the other organs. The veins are seen springing or continuing from these extreme arterial parts, as rivers may be said to spring, and to form at last trunks of large and larger size by which they bring back the blood to the centre of the circulation to be vivified there and carried on again.

From this distribution of blood in these minute vessels the structures of organs derive their constituent parts; through these vessels brain matter,

muscle, gland, membrane is given out from the
blood by a refined process of selection of material,
which, up to this time, is only so far understood as
to enable us to say that it exists.

The minute and intermediate vessels are more
intimately connected than any other part with the
construction and with the function of the living
matter of which the body is composed. Think
you that this mechanism is left uncontrolled?
No; the vessels, small as they are, are under distinct control. Infinitely refined in structure, they
nevertheless have the power of contraction and
dilatation, which power is governed by nervous
action of a special kind. If we pass to the lower
class of animals, we find, running along the body,
in addition to its vascular system, a series of
points of nervous matter, consisting of what are
called ganglia. These ganglia are connected together in chain, and from them filaments of nerves
emanate, which are distributed to all the active
moving parts of the body. In such lower animals
the nervous system thus described stands alone,
and when we rise in the scale and come even to
man we find still the same primitive nervous chain.
But we find also now another and more highly developed nervous system, the centres of which are
locked up in the brain and spinal column, from
which centres nerves of special sense go into the
organs of sense, nerves of sensibility or common
sensation go to the skin and other sensitive surfaces, and nerves of voluntary motion go to the
muscles, all combining to perform their respective
functions in the animal economy.

Thus man has two nervous systems : the primary nervous chain and the added centres, with their fibres. The two systems are connected by their fibres in different parts, but they are still distinct, both anatomically and functionally. The primary nervous system is called the system of the organic vegetative or animal life ; it governs all those motions which are purely involuntary, and its centres are believed by some, and I think with perfect correctness, to be the seats of those faculties which we call emotional and instinctive. The centres of the brain and spinal cord, with their parts, are the centres of the motor and volitional and of the reasoning powers ; of all those faculties, that is to say, which are directly under the influence of the will.

Keep in mind, if you please, the two nervous systems, and add to the remembrance this one additional fact, that all those minute blood-vessels at the extremities of the circulation are under the control of the primary or organic nervous supply. Branches of nerves from those organic centres accompany every arterial vessel throughout the body to its termination, and without direction from our will regulate the contraction and dilation of the blood-vessels to their most refined distribution. This fact was suspected by the older anatomists, but it remained for modern research to make it a demonstration. Thus it has now been proved that if the organic nervous supply of a part of the minute circulation be cut off by division of the organic nerve feeding that part, the vessels become paralysed, as these flexor muscles of my hand,

which now grasp so firmly, would be paralysed
were their voluntary nervous supply divided.

It will be clear at once that an important advancement of knowledge respecting the course of
the blood through the minute circulation has been
gained; but our knowledge does not rest at this
point. When certain simple physical impressions
are made upon the organic nerves, the disturbance
of their supply is indicated by distant phenomena,
and the blush which mantles, and the pallor which
overspreads the cheek, under the influence of
mental emotion or shock, are phenomena of this
order.

I can bring to your notice an experiment, showing the production of paralysis, and of all the phenomena above quoted by the mere action of cold
upon the organic nervous fibre. By evaporating
ether from the back of my hand quickly, I can
freeze the skin, and thereby produce paralysis. I
take the ether away, and now into the paralysed
vessels, which are capable of offering no efficient
resistance, the blood rushes, distending the vessels, remaining for a moment stagnant in them,
and giving a brilliant red color or crimson blush
over the part. I feel in this part the glow commonly called hot-ache; it is the blush which occurs on the cheek, and it is from the same physiological condition.

Still further in advance, and with the mention
of the fact, I am brought back to the subject
proper of my lecture: we have learned that certain chemical agents can so influence the organic
nervous chain as to disturb its functions, after the

manner of a pure physical act. When the peculiar fluid the nitrite of amyl, to which I have before called your attention, came before me for investigation, I divined, from the symptoms it produced, that it influenced the organic nervous fibre precisely after the manner of a division of that fibre. I dipped a spill of paper into the liquid, brought that near to my nose, inhaled the vapor, and immediately felt my face in a red glow, as you see it again at this moment, and felt my heart beating rapidly, as I feel it beating at the present time. I reasoned, naturally, and as events proved, correctly, that this fluid, by its action on the organic nerves, paralysed the vessels of the minute circulation, and finding this to obtain with one chemical agent I traced it in others, and found a class of chemical substances, all of which have this same property of relaxing the blood-vessels at their extreme parts. The whole series of the nitrites possess this power; ether possesses it; but the great point I want to bring forth from this description is, that the substance we are specially dealing with, alcohol, possesses the self-same power. By this influence it produces all those peculiar effects which in every-day life are so frequently illustrated. It paralyses the minute blood-vessels, and allows them to become dilated with the flowing blood.

If you attend a large dinner party, you will observe after the first few courses, when the wine is beginning to circulate, a progressive change in some of those about you who have taken wine. The face begins to get flushed, the eye brightens,

and the murmur of conversation becomes loud.
What is the reason of that flushing of the countenance? It is the same as the flush from blushing,
or from the reaction of cold, or from the nitrite of
amyl. It is the dilatation of vessels following
upon the reduction of nervous control, which reduction has been induced by the alcohol. In a
word, the first stage, the stage of vascular excitement from alcohol, has been established.

The action of the alcohol extending so far does
not stop there. With the disturbance of power in
the extreme vessels, more disturbance is set up in
other organs, and the first organ that shares in it
is the heart. With each beat of the heart a certain degree of resistance is offered by the vessels
when their nervous supply is perfect, and the
stroke of the heart is moderated in respect both to
tension and to time. But when the vessels are
rendered relaxed, the resistance is removed, the
heart begins to run quicker, like a watch from
which the pallets have been removed, and the
heart-stroke, losing nothing in force, is greatly
increased in frequency, with a weakened recoil
stroke. It is easy to account in this manner for
the quickened heart and pulse which accompany
the first stage of deranged action from alcohol,
and you will be interested to know to what extent
this increase of vascular action proceeds. The information on this point is exceedingly curious and
important. After I had observed the effect of
alcohol on the circulation generally, I attempted
to calculate the rate at which it expedited the
rate of circulation by observing its effect on the

beat of the heart in the pigeon. Alcohol may be administered to this bird quite painlessly, and, as the animal quickly goes to sleep under the influence, and is therefore perfectly quiet, the beatings of its heart can be calculated with precision. I traced in these observations an increase of beats of the heart amounting, in the course of two hours, to one-fourth beyond what was natural. Then I essayed to make researches on myself, but many circumstances intervened, connected with the persistent labor and anxiety of professional life, which prevented me conducting the necessary operations so correctly as I desired, and as I might perhaps at another time have done. Fortunately, the information has been far more ably supplied by the researches of Dr. Parkes, of Netley, and the late Count Wollowicz. The researches of these distinguished inquirers are so valuable I make no apology for giving them in detail. The observers conducted their inquiries on the young and healthy adult man. They counted the beats of the heart, first at regular intervals, during what were called water periods, that is to say, periods when the subject under observation drank nothing but water; and next, taking still the same subject, they counted the beats of the heart during successive periods in which alcohol was taken in increasing quantities. Thus step by step they measured the precise action of alcohol on the heart, and thereby the precise primary influence induced by alcohol. The results are stated by themselves as follows:—

The average number of beats of the heart in 24 hours (as calculated from eight observations made in 14 hours), during the first, or water period, was 106,000; in the earlier alcoholic period it was 127,000 or about 21,000 more; and in the later period it was 131,000 or 25,000 more.

"The highest of the daily means of the pulse observed during the first or water period was 77.5; but on this day two observations are deficient. The next highest daily mean was 77 beats.

"If, instead of the mean of the eight days, or 73.57, we compare the mean of this one day, viz., 77 beats per minute, with the alcoholic days, so as to be sure not to over-estimate the action of the alcohol, we find :—

"On the 9th day, with one fluid ounce of alcohol, the heart beat 4,300 times more.

"On the 10th day, with two fluid ounces, 8,172 times more.

"On the 11th day, with four fluid ounces, 12,960 times more.

"On the 12th day, with six fluid ounces, 30,672 times more.

"On the 13th day, with eight fluid ounces, 23,904 times more.

"On the 14th day, with eight fluid ounces, 25,488 times more.

"But as there was ephemeral fever on the 12th day, it is right to make a deduction, and to estimate the number of beats in that day as midway between the 11th and 13th days, or 18,432. Adopting this, the mean daily excess of beats during the alcoholic days was 14,492, or an increase of rather more than 13 per cent.

"The first day of alcohol gave an excess of 4

per cent., and the last of 23 per cent.; and the
mean of these two gives almost the same percentage of excess as the mean of the six days.

" Admitting that each beat of the heart was as
strong during the alcoholic period as in the water
period (and it was really more powerful), the heart
on the last two days of alcohol was doing one-
fifth more work.

" Adopting the lowest estimate which has been
given of the daily work of the heart, viz., as equal
to 122 tons lifted one foot, the heart during the
alcoholic period did daily work in excess equal to
lifting 15.8 tons one foot, and in the last two days
did extra work to the amount of 24 tons lifted
as far.

" The period of rest for the heart was shortened, though, perhaps, not to such an extent as
would be inferred from the number of beats, for
each contraction was sooner over. The heart, on
the fifth and sixth days after alcohol was left off,
and apparently at the time when the last traces of
alcohol were eliminated, showed in the sphygmo-
graphic tracings signs of unusual feebleness; and,
perhaps, in consequence of this, when the brandy
quickened the heart again, the tracings showed a
more rapid contraction of the ventricles, but less
power than in the alcoholic period. The brandy
acted, in fact, on a heart whose nutrition had not
been perfectly restored."

It will seem at first sight almost incredible that
such an excess of work could be put upon the
heart, but it is perfectly credible when all the
facts are known. The heart of an adult man

makes, as we see above, 73.57 strokes per minute.
This number multiplied by sixty for the hour, and
again by twenty-four hours for the entire day,
would give nearly 106,000 as the number of strokes
per day. There is, however, a reduction of stroke
produced by assuming the recumbent position and
by sleep, so that for simplicity's sake we may take
off the 6,000 strokes, and speaking generally may
put the average at 100,000 in the entire day. With
each of these strokes the two ventricles of the
heart, as they contract, lift up into their respective
vessels three ounces of blood each, that is to say,
six ounces with the combined stroke, or 600,000 in
the twenty-four hours. The equivalent of work
rendered by this simpler calculation would be 116
foot tons; and if we estimate the increase of work
induced by alcohol we shall find that four ounces
of spirit increase it one-eighth part; six ounces,
one-sixth part; and eight ounces, one-fourth part.

The stage of primary excitement of the circulation thus induced lasts for a considerable time, but
at length the heart flags from its over action, and
requires the stimulus of more spirit to carry it on
in its work. Let us take what we may call a moderate amount of alcohol, say two ounces by volume, in form of wine, or beer, or spirits. What is
called strong sherry or port may contain as much
as twenty-five per cent. by volume. Brandy over
fifty; gin, thirty-eight; rum, forty-eight; whisky,
forty-three; vin ordinaire, eight; strong ale, fourteen; champagne, ten to eleven; it matters not
which, if the quantity of alcohol be regulated by
the amount present in the liquor imbibed. When

we reach the two ounces, a distinct physiological effect follows, leading on to that first stage of excitement with which we are now conversant. The reception of the spirit arrested at this point, there need be no important mischief done to the organism; but if the quantity imbibed be increased, further changes quickly occur. We have seen that all the organs of the body are built upon the vascular structures, and therefore it follows that a prolonged paralysis of the minute circulation must of necessity lead to disturbance in other organs than the heart.

By common observation the flush seen on the cheek during the first stage of alcoholic excitation is presumed to extend merely to the parts actually exposed to view. It cannot, however, be too forcibly impressed that the condition is universal in the body. If the lungs could be seen, they too would be found with their vessels injected; if the brain and spinal cord could be laid open to view, they would be discovered in the same condition; if the stomach, the liver, the spleen, the kidneys, or any other vascular organs or parts could be exposed, the vascular engorgement would be equally manifest. In the lower animals I have been able to witness this extreme vascular condition in the lungs, and there are here presented to you two drawings from nature, showing, one the lungs in a natural state of an animal killed by a sudden blow, the other the lungs of an animal killed equally suddenly, but at a time when it was under the influence of alcohol. You will see, as if you were looking at the structures themselves, how different they are in respect to the blood which they contained, how intensely charged with blood is the lung in which the vessels had been paralysed by the alcoholic spirit.

I once had the unusual, though unhappy, opportunity of observing the same phenomenon in the brain structure of a man who, in a paroxysm of alcoholic excitement, decapitated himself under the wheel of a railway carriage, and whose brain was instantaneously evolved from the skull by the crash. The brain itself, entire, was before me within three minutes after the death. It exhaled the odor of spirit most distinctly, and its membranes and minute structures were vascular in the extreme. It looked as if it had been recently injected with vermilion. The white matter of the cerebrum, studded with red points, could scarcely be distinguished, when it was incised, by its natural whiteness; and the pia-mater, or internal vascular membrane covering the brain, resembled a delicate web of coagulated red blood, so tensely were its fine vessels engorged.

I should add that this condition extended through both the larger and the smaller brain, the cerebrum and cerebellum, but was not so marked in the medulla or commencing portion of the spinal cord.

The action of alcohol continued beyond the first stage, the function of the spinal cord is influenced. Through this part of the nervous system we are accustomed, in health, to perform automatic acts of a mechanical kind, which proceed systematically even when we are thinking or speaking on other subjects. Thus a skilled workman will continue his mechanical work perfectly, while his mind is bent on some other subject ; and thus we all perform various acts in a purely automatic way, without calling in the aid of the higher centres, except something more than ordinary occurs to demand their service, upon which we think before we perform. Under alcohol, as the spinal centres become influenced, these pure automatic acts cease to be correctly carried on. That the hand may reach any object, or the foot be correctly planted, the higher intellectual centre must be invoked to make the proceeding secure. There follows quickly upon this a deficient power of co-ordination of muscular movement. The nervous control of certain of the muscles is lost, and the nervous stimulus is more or less enfeebled. The muscles of the lower lip in the human subject usually fail first of all, then the muscles of the lower limbs, and it is worthy of remark that the extensor muscles give way earlier than the flexors. The muscles themselves by this time are also failing in power; they respond more feebly than is natural to the nervous stimulus; they, too, are coming under the depressing influence of the paralysing agent, their structure is temporarily deranged, and their contractile power reduced.

This modification of the animal functions under alcohol marks the second degree of its action. In young subjects there is now, usually, vomiting with faintness, followed by gradual relief from the burden of the poison.

The alcoholic spirit carried yet a further degree,

the cerebral or brain centres become influenced; they are reduced in power, and the controlling influences of will and of judgment are lost. As these centres are unbalanced and thrown into chaos, the rational part of the nature of the man gives way before the emotional, passional, or organic part. The reason is now off duty, or is fooling with duty, and all the mere animal instincts and sentiments are laid atrociously bare. The coward shows up more craven, the braggart more boastful, the cruel more merciless, the untruthful more false, the carnal more degraded. "*In vino veritas*" expresses, even indeed to physiological accuracy, the true condition. The reason, the emotions, the instincts, are all in a state of carnival, and in chaotic feebleness.

Finally, the action of the alcohol still extending, the superior brain centres are overpowered; the senses are beclouded, the voluntary muscular prostration is perfected, sensibility is lost, and the body lies a mere log, dead by all but one-fourth, on which alone its life hangs. The heart still remains true to its duty, and while it just lives it feeds the breathing power. And so the circulation and the respiration, in the otherwise inert mass, keeps the mass within the bare domain of life until the poison begins to pass away and the nervous centres to revive again. It is happy for the inebriate that, as a rule, the brain fails so long before the heart that he has neither the power nor the sense to continue his process of destruction up to the act of death of his circulation. Therefore he lives to die another day.

Thus there are four stages of alcoholic action in

the primary form :— (*a*) A stage of vascular excitement and exhaustion ; (*b*) a stage of excitement and exhaustion of the spinal cord, with muscular perturbation ; (*c*) a stage of unbalanced reasoning power and of volition ; (*d*) a stage of complete collapse of nervous function.

Such is an outline of the primary action of alcohol on those who may be said to be unaccustomed to it, or who have not yet fallen into a fixed habit of taking it. For a long time the organism will bear these perversions of its functions without apparent injury, but if the experiment be repeated too often and too long, if it be continued after the term of life when the body is fully developed, when the elasticity of the membranes and of the blood vessels is lessened, and when the tone of the muscular fibre is reduced, then organic series of structural changes, so characteristic of the persistent effects of spirit, become prominent and permanent. Then the external surface becomes darkened and congested, its vessels, in parts, visibly large ; the skin becomes blotched, the proverbial red nose is defined, and those other striking vascular changes which disfigure many who may probably be called moderate alcoholics, are developed. These changes, belonging as they do to external surfaces, come under direct observation ; they are accompanied with certain other changes in the internal organs, which we shall discover in a future lecture to be more destructive still.

LECTURE IV.

THE question that lies before us for discussion
in this lecture is short and definite.   It is included
in the three words: Is alcohol food?

We have studied in the previous lecture the
purely physical action of alcohol on the animal
body, that which stands apart from the action of
food, and we have learned from the study that over
the nervous system and over the vascular supply
this spirit exerts a specific influence.   We now inquire whether the influence ends there, or whether
there may be, in addition, either a sustaining, and
constructing, or a heat-giving power—that is to
say, a force-giving quality in it.   If there be, then
the simple physical effects are perchance tolerable,
or at all events are not sufficient to militate against
the advantages which lie on the food side of the
question.

It may be well to rest for a moment to consider
the position of men and animals upon the earth in
relation to the means given to them for their support as living, moving, and, in the higher animals,
thinking structures.   This position is well-defined.
The theory that man was made originally out of
the dust of the earth is, after all, the most scientific

theory that has ever been advanced as to his primeval origin, if the word *dust* be only extended so as to include the actual compound substance of the earth. For in the earth are to be found not only all the elements out of which he is constructed, but even certain of the elements in the same kind of combination as we find them in him. In the earth water, salts, and organic matter are found ; in man the same are found. The man is in many respects of motion a reflex of the motion of the earth, presenting periodicities of movements, and of movements in a circle in like mode. As if to complete the analogy, this remains true, that the earth yields spontaneously to man, either from herself directly or from the vegetable kingdom which lies between her and man, all the requirements for his existence. Whatever, therefore, man invents, though it may seem to be a great necessity, is not a necessity except to those who, being trained to its use, have been led artificially to believe it essential. Thus nature has produced water and milk for man to drink, and they are, in truth, all the fluids that are essential. This lesson, which nature teaches by her rule of provision for the necessities of animal life, is supplemented by many other facts, each equally authoritative. There is ever before us the great experiment that all classes of living beings beneath man require as drink none other fluids except those I have named. We see the most useful of these animals performing laborious tasks, undergoing extremes of fatigue, bearing vicissitudes of heat and of cold, and enduring work, fatigue, and vicissitude for long series of

years, sustained by their solid food, with no other
fluid than simple water. We see again whole
nations and races of men who labor hard, endure
fatigue and exposure, and who live to the end of a
long and healthy life, taking with their solid sustenance water only as a beverage.

When we turn to the physiological construction
either of man or of a lower animal, we discover
nothing that can lead us to conceive the necessity
for any other fluid than that which nature has
supplied. The mass of the blood is composed of
water, the mass of the nervous system is composed
of water, the mass of all the active vital organs is
made up of the same fluid : the secretions are
watery fluids, and if in any of these parts any
other agent than water should replace it, the result is an instant disturbance of function that is
injurious in proportion to the displacement.

When we turn therefore to the use of such a
fluid as alcohol under any of its disguises—as spirit,
as wine, as beer, as cider, as perry, as liqueur,—
we are driven *à priori* to look upon it as something
superadded to the necessities of life ; to look upon
it, in a word, as a luxury. In such sense it has
always been received amongst those nations which
have most indulged in it. It is something added
to the ordinary life ; something unnecessary, but
agreeable. Wine, added to the meal, transforms
the meal into a feast ; it is supposed to make glad
the heart, but it is never supposed that if the wine
were not possessed the life would be shortened.
When now we offer wine, it is, by the effect of
habit and education, an offering of a thing that is

super-necessitous, and in such wise a compliment, an indication of desire or of willingness to be exceedingly hospitable.

All the evidence of a general kind which can be gathered from these observations points to the uselessness, for man, of such an artificial agent as alcohol. But, after all, an assumption so derived may be false. We have already seen that when alcoholic spirit is taken into the animal body it produces in it exceedingly marked effects; it may therefore, by accident, I might almost say, play in some manner the part of a food and supplement water. Indeed, it is a form of water in which a compound of carbon and hydrogen has replaced hydrogen. Let us, then, ask the question : Can alcohol be in any sense accepted as performing any other part in the body save that physical part which we have considered? Can it have happened that man, by his invention, has added, to nature, a food? And let us answer the question as candidly as the facts of experiment and experience will permit.

CONSTRUCTIVE MATERIALS OF THE BODY.

The living animal body is constructed out of a few simple forms of matter which possess, during life, the power of motion. It is, in its living state, a noun and a verb. Whatever helps to maintain it in perfect order of construction, whatever enables it to move of its own mere will and motion, may be considered as a food. The one gives matter and mass, the other gives force or spirit to the mass. With the progress of organic chemistry, after the discovery of the art of organic analysis, it soon became evident that what are called foods are divisible into two great classes; those which supply material or tissue, and those which supply heat or other variety of force. Gradually it was detected that the building foods all contain the element nitrogen as an essential part, and that the force-supplying foods are free of nitrogen and are hydro-carbons, substances that will undergo combustion by oxidation, and liberate force for the motive uses of the economy. So, foods have for a long time been sharply classified as nitrogenous or tissue-feeding, and as respiratory or heat-producing. At the present moment this long accepted view is undergoing some modification. It is being elicited that the nitrogenous foods are to a certain degree heat-producing; but I need not at this stage enter on the nice question involved. I may safely, for the practical purpose we have in view, let the division of the classes of foods remain as described above.

The nitrogenous foods exist in the animal body in the form of what is called colloidal matter, the word *colloidal* being a term signifying a jelly-like substance. The purest form of this matter is found in the blood in the white, elastic, plastic matter, called fibrine. By repeated washings of a portion of this substance, I have prepared here, from the blood of the ox, a beautiful specimen of this colloid of the blood. Of a similar colloidal substance the moving muscles are formed. In a fluid state, and permanently fluid at the temperature of the living body, the colloid called albumen forms part

of organic structure. Under the names of gela-
tine and chondrine, a nitrogenous colloidal substance forms the organic matter of the skeleton,
of the cartilages, of the sheaths of muscles, of the
tendons. The eye-ball is constructed out of a
series of colloidal tissues. All the membranes
which envelope the visceral organs, and which
possess elasticity, are colloidal. The outer covering or skin is colloidal, the nails are the same.
Even in the brain and nervous matter there is distributed a colloid. Thus, if we sum up the various
parts of the body we may say that all the active
masses of structure are nitrogenous and colloidal.

In combination with this active matter there are,
however, two other material ingredients, viz., water
and saline substance. Upon its combination with
water the activity of the colloid depends. Upon
the saline rests the various kinds of combination
of the colloid with the water. In bone the gela-
tine is combined with a salt, called phosphate of
lime, with carbonate of lime, and other salts, in
much larger proportion than itself. In fibrine the
colloidal substance is nearly divested of saline;
but in all parts these three material compounds
make up the animal structures.

Lying outside these structures in the natural
state, but really as an adventitious formation, is
one other animal product, viz., fat; a substance
detrimental to the motion of the active parts when
present in excess, but at the same time capable of
combustion, and of yielding heat by the process.

We have now before us the constructive or
building parts of the animal body. Excepting the

water, the salts, and the fat, they all contain nitrogen, and they take their specific quality from that
specific fact. We know that the source of them is
the vegetable kingdom, that they are formed by
nature in that kingdom, are transferred from the
vegetable to the animal, are not made by any natural process within the animal, have not yet been
made by any artificial process known to the chemist, and can therefore only be supplied from the
one natural supply.

Alcohol contains no nitrogen, it has none of the
qualities of these structure-building foods; it is
incapable of being transformed into any of them;
it is therefore not a food in the sense of its being
a constructive agent in the building up of the body.

In respect to this view there is, I believe, now
no difference of opinion amongst those who have
most carefully observed the action of alcohol.
There is, however, a difference in relation to its
action as a fat-forming food. It appears to be on
evidence that men and animals beginning, while
in a perfect state of health, to take in excess certain fluids containing alcohol become fattened.
Notoriously, ale and beer fatten; and in some
parts of the country certain animals—calves, for
instance—are rapidly fattened by the process of
feeding them with a mixture of barley flour and
gin. But through all these apparent evidences
there may run an error. The fattening may not
be due to the alcohol itself, but to the sugar or the
starchy material that is taken with it. As a matter of general experience on which I have tried
to arrive at the truth with as much accuracy as

can be obtained, I am led to the conclusion that pure spirit drinkers among men, I mean those who do not mix sugar with the spirit, and who dislike spirit which is artificially sweetened, are not fattened by the spirit they take. This tallies also with the observations on the action of absolute alcohol on inferior animals, for they certainly, under that influence, if they are allowed liberty to move freely, do not fatten.

The question of the effect of alcohol in fattening presents still another difficulty. Alcohol, when it is largely taken, unless the will of the imbiber be very powerful, is wont to induce desire for undue sleep, or at least desire for physical repose. Under such conditions there is an interference with the ordinary nutritive processes. The wasted products of nutrition are imperfectly eliminated, the respiration becomes slower and less effective, and there is set up a series of changes leading, independently of the alcohol as a direct producer of fat, to development and to deposit of fatty tissue in the body. All these circumstances militate against the hypothesis of the origin of fatty material direct from alcohol, nor is there any obvious chemical fact that supports the hypothesis. We understand chemically the transformation of starchy matter into one form of sugar, and we infer that in the animal body sugar is transmutable into fat. We know also that we can transmute sugar into alcohol, but as yet we see no way back from alcohol into sugar; if we did, the difficulty of tracing alcohol into fat would probably be over.

Physiological argument nevertheless lends some countenance to the view that alcohol may, by an unknown process, be transferable into fat. It is true that some confirmed alcoholics who do not wax fat in the ordinary sense of the term, that is to say, who do not fill out with fat, from the separation of fatty matter in their cellular tissue outside the vital organs, do, in certain instances, undergo a process of fatty change within their organic structures. Their muscles, including the heart, become the centres of the degeneration called "fatty," and by the interposition of cells of fat in the minute muscular elements, the activity of the fabric is destroyed, sometimes to a fatal destruction. The same degenerative change may extend also to other organs, to the brain and to such active glands as the liver and the kidney.

At first view it occurs to the mind that here is evidence of effect upon cause. At the same time it is not so clear that the effect is direct from alcohol; for when we proceed to examine into all the data that lie before us, we discover such an absence of uniformity in differing examples of the fatty change that we lose alcohol as the clue to discovery. Some alcoholics truly present the fatty modification of tissue, other alcoholics do not present it, so that alcohol may be in active operation and may neither be promoting the production of fat from other material nor yielding it. Lastly, the fatty change of tissue may progress, in the absence of alcohol, in the tissues of those who altogether abstain.

In conclusion, therefore, on this one point of alcohol, its use as a builder of the substantial parts of the animal organism, I fear I must give up all hope of affirmative proof. It does not certainly help to build up the active nitrogenous structures. It probably does not produce fatty matter, except by an indirect and injurious interference with the natural processes.

If alcohol be not a substance out of which the animal tissues are formed, may it not be a source of energy of actual motion ; may it not supply the power of doing work? Alcohol, we see, contains two elements that will burn in the presence of oxygen, viz., carbon and hydrogen, and although by their combination already with oxygen in the alcohol a certain measure of their potential energy is lost, they are still capable of combining with more oxygen. This is proved by various experiments. When alcohol is burned, that is to say, when its combustible elements combine with free oxygen, there results from the chemical combination a certain degree of heat. The heat produced does not approach that obtained by an equal weight of hydrogen, it is not so great as that produced by an equal weight of carbon, but it is greater than that caused by the combustion of phosphorus, and very much greater than that caused by the combustion of sulphur.

The combustion thus spoken of is that active combustion which is excited when a light is brought into contact with alcohol so that its vapor may burn. But it is not actually necessary that such instant active combustion should be set up. If we distribute alcohol over a wide surface in the presence of some chemical substances it will then by its combination with oxygen liberate a greater or lesser degree of heat. If we saturate a portion of paper with alcohol, and on that paper pour a little of the finely-divided powder called platinum black, we at once get evidence of heat which may be so active that perfect combustion may ensue. In this instance the alcohol is transformed, as in burning, in great part, nay it may be altogether, into carbonic acid and water, which means the completed combustion. If in place of absolute alcohol, in this experiment, we were to use alcohol diluted with water, then instead of obtaining the active combination and combustion we should get a slower oxidation with the production of substances to which attention has already been directed, viz., aldehyde, acetic acid, and volatile acetic ether.

DISPOSAL OF ALCOHOL IN THE ORGANISM.

We are brought now to one of the most important parts of our study. We see that, under favoring conditions, alcohol will oxidise in the presence of the air. We see that it will oxidise in two ways—actively, with the production of much heat and with the formation of carbonic acid and water; passively, with the production of aldehyde and acetic acid.

In the human body do any similar changes take place? Throughout the whole of the vast sheet of the minute circulation there is ever in progress, during life, a process of slow oxidation of carbon and hydrogen, by which heat is produced, and carbonic acid and water are produced. The heat is proved by the animal warmth which is ever present in our bodies while we live; the carbonic acid and water, as products, are proved by their continued presence in the secretions from the lungs, skin, and other organs.

Alcohol, we have seen, is carried by the blood into this minute circulation. Is it possible it can pass through that ordeal and undergo no chemical change? If it does undergo any change, what is its nature? These questions have occupied the attention of many gifted minds; but they are not yet solved. Let me endeavor to put the position in which they stand plainly before you.

The earlier physiologists of this century came, naturally enough, to the conclusion that the alcohol taken into the body is consumed there with the evolution of heat. A certain development of heat in the superficies of the body, and a certain sensation of glow which follows upon the imbibition of spirit lent countenance to this suspicion. But in course of time, independently of any knowledge of the effect produced by alcohol in the minute circulation of the blood, it began to be doubted whether alcohol was disposed of in the organism by its combustion. Some observers had noticed, in conducting the examination of the body after death from excess of alcohol, that the odor of the substance was present in the tissues, especially in the nervous tissue, and it was doubted whether the alcohol might not under some circumstances remain in the organism without

undergoing any change at all. In 1860 two eminent Frenchmen—Lallemand and Perrin, assisted
by Duroy, published a prize essay on alcohol, in
which this view was maintained, or, as the authors
would probably say, was originated ; for in truth
they were the first to state the view on direct
scientific evidence. From the result of many experiments, they came to the conclusion that
alcohol taken into the living body accumulates
in the tissues, especially in the liver and in the
brain, and that it is eliminated by the fluid secretions, notably by the renal secretion, as alcohol.
They sought in the different tissues for evidence
of the secondary products of the oxidation of
alcohol, for aldehyde, acetal, acetic acid, and they
found none of those products, except some acetic
acid in the stomach, which acid they concluded
was formed from the alcohol received directly
into the stomach, and from the action exerted
upon it there by the gastric juice. The experiments carried on by these inquirers were so
numerous and careful, and the results they arriv-
ed at were so definitely stated, that their labors
were for a season accepted as conclusive by many
men of science, and by the majority of the public.
It was ascertained by other experimentalists that
alcohol is eliminated by the system in the direct
way, as alcohol, and the question of elimination
rested as if it had been solved.

The interval of credence in these assertions was
not very prolonged. An English physician soon
commenced to cross a lance with his learned
French peers, and to point out certain distinct

errors in their results. I have no doubt many of you know, before I mention his name, that he to whom I refer was the physician who last year lost his life from the performance of his professional duties—the late Dr. Anstie. Respecting this observer, whose friendship I owned for many years, it is meet for me to pay this public tribute of respect; that no man I ever knew combined with vigor of mind, more incomparable industry and courage, or a more honorable regard for scientific truth and honesty. The subject we are now considering has lost no investigator more ably learned for the work that still remains to be done.

From Dr. Anstie came the earliest expressions of doubt relative to this hypothesis of what is called the direct elimination of alcohol by the secretions, and from him have come the latest objections. His arguments have been sustained abroad by Schulinus, and, in this country, by Drs. Thudichum and Dupré, whose work on wine will, even in another century, be more highly prized, if that be possible, than it is now. The sum and substance of the labors of these observers is stated in a few words. They prove that while it is true that, under certain circumstances, alcohol taken into the body will pass off in the secretions unchanged, the quantity so eliminated is the merest fraction of what has been injected, and that there must be some other means by which the spirit is disposed of in the organism. In a lecture I delivered on this subject in the year 1869, I ventured to suggest, in commenting upon a series of Dr. Thudichum's remarkable researches, that perhaps one

element of research was wanting to prove conclusively the fallacy of the direct elimination hypothesis. I thought that sufficient time had not
been allowed between the administration of the
spirit and the final determination made for it in the
excreted fluids. It was not, I argued, shown how
much spirit the tissues would hold unchanged.
The objection was sound, but it has been removed
by more recent experiment.

In the last research conducted by Anstie, in
which he was assisted by Dupré, the results of the
experiments were unmistakable in their bearing on
the points now under our consideration. The history of these labors is recorded in full in the last
paper written by Dr. Anstie, and published in the
journal called the *Practitioner*, for July, 1874.

The test that had been commonly employed for
determining the presence of alcohol in the fluid
suspected of containing it, was the color test. A
solution is made consisting of bichromate of potassa, with diluted sulphuric acid. When to this
solution alcohol is added, there is a change of
color from the brownish red to green; owing to
the reduction of the chromic acid to the green
oxide of the base chromium. By marking the
difference of color produced a scale can be adopted
which will show the extent of the reduction, and
thereby the amount of the spirit that has caused
the change. This process was improved by Dr.
Dupré. He distilled the fluid in which alcohol
was believed to be present, and then, after treating
the distillate with the bichromate and sulphuric
acid solution, he tested with a standard solution

of soda for the amount of acetic acid which would be produced by the oxidation of alcohol were that fluid present.

This modification of test was and is a very considerable advance, since it enabled the observers to extend their determinations with greater accuracy of detail. In the research they conducted with it two facts of singular interest were elicited. The first fact was discovered by Dr. Dupré. It is that from the secretions of persons who do not drink alcohol at all a fluid can be distilled which affects the chromic test as if alcohol were actually present in the secreted fluids, and that this hitherto unsuspected product is oxidised into an acid so like acetic acid it cannot be distinguished from it, and is apparently identical with it. To be plain, Dr. Dupré's discovery suggests that no man can be, in strict scientific sense, a non-alcoholic, inasmuch as, " will he nill he," he brews in his own economy a "wee drap." It is an innocent brew certainly, but it is brewed, and the most ardent abstainer must excuse it. " Argal, he that is not guilty of his own death shorteneth not his own life." The fault, if it be one, rests with nature, who, according to our poor estimates, is no more faultless than the rest of her sex.

The second fact, which came chiefly from the labors of Dr. Anstie, is that from animals under alcohol, not one of the secretions, not all the secretions combined, yield any more than a fractional amount of the alcohol that has been administered. The experiments were by necessity made on the inferior animals, but they supplied none the less conclusively the fact stated. It was proved that an animal, a terrier dog, weighing ten pounds, could take with comparative impunity nearly 2000 grains of absolute alcohol in ten days, and that on the last day of this regimen he only eliminated by all the channels of elimination 1.13 grains of alcohol. This fact was of itself sufficiently remarkable, but another still more important remains to be told. In completion of his research, when an animal had been treated with alcohol, as above described, Anstie killed it, instantly and painlessly, two hours after it had received the last quantity— 95 grains—of spirit. Then the whole body, including every fragment of tissue with all the fluid and solid contents, was subjected to analysis, with the result of discovering only 23.66 grains of spirit.

We are driven by the evidence now before us to the certain conclusion that in the animal body alcohol is decomposed; that is to say, a certain portion of it (and if a certain portion why not the whole?) is transmutable into new compounds. The inference that might be drawn is fair enough that the alcohol is lost by being burned in the body. It is lost in the body, and out of the body it will burn. If it will burn in the organism it will supply force, for it enters as the bearer of so much potential energy. In combining with oxygen is there then a development of force or heat to the extent that would be developed in the combustion of the same quantity in the lamp, or from the distribution of it over the platinum black? At the same time, and in corroboration, is the product of its combustion, carbonic acid, to be discovered in the excretions? If there be heat, and if there be product of carbon consumed in oxygen, then alcohol must rank as a heat-forming food.

DOES ALCOHOL CAUSE INCREASE OF ANIMAL HEAT?

In putting before you this inquiry, I am prepared to answer it by direct knowledge gained from individual experiment. In the course of some researches I had to make for reports rendered to the British Association for the Advancement of Science, it became part of my duty to ascertain what effect certain chemical agents exert over the animal temperature. Amongst these agents was alcohol.

At the time when my researches commenced—viz., in the year 1864, there was nothing definitely known on the subject. The thermometer was not then in such general use as it is now, and it had not been applied, as far as I know, to this particular determination. Generally, however, it had been assumed by the majority of persons that alcohol warms the body, and to " take just a drop to keep out the cold " had been the practice which the experience of ages seemed to justify. It is fair, at the same time, to say that Dr. Lees, and some other far-seeing observers, had for many years held and asserted a different view. They had not entered into minuteness of experimental detail, but they had observed from the effects of alcohol on those who had been exposed to cold in the extreme North and in other regions of ice and snow, that the drinkers did not live on like other men. Thus, in so far as I had what is called experience to guide me, I found conflict of opinion. It was not my business, however, to accept guidance of this kind, but to appeal to the only safe guide, the direct interrogation of nature by experiment.

It were impossible for me to recount the details of the long research,—extending, with intervals of rest, over three years,—which was conducted in my laboratory, to determine the influence of alcohol on the animal temperature. The effects were observed on warm-blooded animals of different kinds, including birds; on the human subject in health, and on the same subject under alcoholic disease. Similar experiments were made in different external temperatures of the air, ranging from summer heat to ten degrees below freezing point. The whole were carried on from experiment to experiment, without regard either to comparison or result until the general character of result began to proclaim that a rule existed which could rarely be considered exceptional. The facts obtained I may epitomise as follows:

The progressive stages of change of animal function from alcohol are four in number. The first is a stage of excitement when there exists that relaxation and injection of the blood-vessels of the minute circulation with which we have become conversant. The second is the stage of excitement with some muscular inability and deficient automatic control. The third is a stage of rambling, incoherent, emotional excitement, with loss of voluntary muscular power, and ending in helpless unconsciousness. The fourth and final stage is that in which the heart itself begins to fail, and in which death, in extreme instances of intoxication, closes the scene. These stages are developed in all the warm-blooded animals, and the changes of temperature throughout the whole are relatively the same.

In the first stage the external temperature of the body is raised. In birds—pigeons—the rise may amount to a full degree, on Fahrenheit's scale; in mammals it rarely exceeds half a degree. In man it may rise to half a degree, and in the confirmed inebriate, in whom the cutaneous vessels are readily engorged, I have seen it run up to a degree and a half. In this stage the effect on the extremities of the nerves is that of a warm glow, like what is experienced during the reaction from cold.

The heat felt in this stage might be considered as due to the combustion of the alcohol: it is not so; it is in truth a process of cooling. It is from the unfolding of the larger sheet of the warm blood and from the quicker radiation of heat from that larger surface. During this stage, which is comparatively brief, the internal temperature is declining; the expired air from the lungs is indicating, not an increase, but the first period of reduction in the amount of carbonic acid, and the reddened surface of the body is so reduced in tonicity that cold applied to it increases the suffusion. It is this most deceptive stage that led the older observers into the error that alcohol warms the body

In the second stage, the temperature first comes down to its natural standard, and then declines below what is natural. The fall is not considerable. In birds it reaches from one and a half to two degrees. In other animals, dogs and guinea pigs, it rarely exceeds one degree; in man it is confined to three-fourths of a degree. In a room heated to 65° or 70° the decrease of animal temperature may not actually be perceived; but it is quickly detected if the person in whom it is present pass into a colder atmosphere, and it lasts, even when the further supply of alcohol is cut off, for a long period—viz., from two and a half to three hours. It is much prolonged by absence of food.

During the third degree the fall of temperature rapidly increases, and as the fourth stage is approached it reaches a decline that becomes actually dangerous. In birds the reduction may be five degrees and a half, and in the other animals three. In man it is often from two and a half to three degrees. There is always during this stage a profound sleep or coma, and while this lasts the temperature continues reduced.

It is here worthy of incidental notice that, as a rule, the sleep of apoplexy and the sleep of drunkenness may be distinguished by a marked difference in the animal temperature. In apoplexy the temperature of the body is above, in drunkenness below, the natural standard of 98° of Fahrenheit's scale.

Under favorable circumstances a long period is required before the body recovers its natural warmth after such reduction of heat as follows the extreme stage of alcoholic intoxication. With the first conscious movements of recovery there is a faint rise, but such is the depression that these very movements exhaust and lead to a further reduction. I have known as long a period as three days required, in man, to bring back a steady natural return of the full animal warmth.

Through every stage, then, of the action of alcohol—barring that first stage of excitement—I found a reduction of animal heat to be the special action of the poison. To make the research more perfectly reliable, I combined the action of alcohol with that of cold. A warm-blooded animal, insensibly asleep in the third stage of alcoholic narcotism, was placed in a chamber, the air of which was reduced in temperature to ten degrees below freezing point, together with another similar animal which had received no alcohol. I found that both sleep under these circumstances, but the alcoholic sleeps to die; the other sleeps more deeply than is natural, and lives so long as the store of food it is charged with continues to support life. Within this bound it awakes, in a warmer air, uninjured, though the degree of cold be carried even lower, and be continued for a much longer time.

One more portion of evidence completes the research on the influence of alcohol on the animal temperature. As there is a decrease of temperature from alcohol, so there is proportionately a decrease in the amount of the natural products of the combustion of the body. The quantity of carbonic acid exhaled by the breath is proportionately diminished with the decline of the animal heat. In the extreme stage of alcoholic insensibility,—short of the actually dangerous,—the amount of carbonic acid exhaled by the animal and given off into the chamber I constructed for the purposes of observation was reduced to one-third below the natural standard. On the human subject in this stage of insensibility the quantity of carbonic acid exhaled has not been measured, but in the earlier stage of alcoholic derangement of function the exhaled gas was measured with much care by a very earnest worker, whose recent death we have also to deplore—Dr. Edward Smith. In these early stages Dr. Smith found that the amount of carbonic acid was reduced in man, as I have found it in the lower animals, so that the fact of the general reduction may be considered as established beyond disputation.

We are landed then at last on this basis of knowledge. An agent that will burn and give forth heat and product of combustion outside the body, and which is obviously decomposed within the body, reduces the animal temperature, and prevents the yield of so much product of combustion as is actually natural to the organic life.

What is the inference? The inference is that the alcohol is not burned after the manner of a food which supports animal combustion ; but that it is decomposed into secondary products, by oxidation, at the expense of the oxygen which ought to be applied for the natural heating of the body.

For some time to come the physiological world

will be studiously intent on the discovery of the mode by which alcohol is removed from the organism. It is a subject on which I shall one day be able to speak, I hope, with some degree of experimental certainty, but on which at this moment I am not prepared to offer more than an indication of the probable course of research. I may venture to add, in advance, two or three suggestions to which my researches, as far as they go, point.

Firstly, I believe there is a certain determinable degree of saturation of the blood with alcohol, within which degree all the alcohol is disposed of by its decomposition. Beyond that degree the oxidation is arrested, and then there is an accumulation of alcohol, with voidance of it, in the unchanged state, in the secretions.

Secondly, the change or decomposition of the alcohol in its course through the minute circulation, in which it is transformed, is not into carbonic acid and water, as though it were burned, but into a new soluble, chemical substance, probably aldehyde, which returns by the veins into the great channels of the circulation.

Thirdly, I think I have made out that there is an outlet for the alcohol, or for the fluid product of its decomposition, into the alimentary canal, through the secretion of the liver. Thrown into the canal, it is, I believe, subjected there to further oxidation, is in fact oxidised by a process of fermentation attended with the active development of gaseous substances. From this surface the oxidised product is in turn re-absorbed in great part and carried into the circulation, and is disposed of by combination with bases or by further oxidation.

Here, however, I leave the theoretical point to revert to the practical, and the practical is this; that alcohol cannot by any ingenuity of excuse for it, be classified amongst the foods of man. It neither supplies matter for construction nor heat. On the contrary, it injures construction and it reduces temperature.

EFFECT OF MUSCULAR POWER.

Behind the question of the effect of alcohol upon the animal temperature was another subject for inquiry. It was fair to ask whether, if heat were not produced by the spirit, some additional stimulus might be communicated by it to the muscular fibre. There is nothing in what we see relating to the action of alcohol in man that would lead us to suppose it capable of giving an increased muscular power, and it is certain that animals subjected even for short periods of time to its influence lose their power for work in a marked degree. Indeed, if we were to treat our domestic animals with this agent in the same manner that we treat ourselves, we should soon have none that were tamable, none that were workable, and none that were edible. I thought it, nevertheless, worth the inquiry whether at any stage of the alcoholic excitement living muscle could be induced to show an extra amount of power. I therefore submitted muscle to this test. I gently weighted the hinder limb of a frog until the power of contraction was just overcome; then by a measured electrical current I stimulated the muscle to extra contraction, and determined the increase of weight that could thus be lifted. This decided upon in the healthy animal, the trial was repeated some days later on the same animal after it had received alcohol in sufficient quantities to induce the various stages of alcoholic modification of function. The result was that through every stage the response to the electrical current was enfeebled, and so soon as narcotism was developed by the spirit, it was so enfeebled that less than half the weight that could be lifted in the previous trial, by the natural effort of the animal, could not now be raised even under the electrical excitation.

In man and in animals, during the period between the first and third stages of alcoholic disturbance, there is often muscular excitement, which passes for increased muscular power. The muscles are then truly more rapidly stimulated into motion by the nervous tumult, but the muscular power is actually enfeebled.

HYGIENIC LESSONS.

The facts I have endeavored to bring forward in this as well as in the last lecture will suggest to the mind many thoughts bearing upon the health of individuals and communities, in so far as health is affected by the potent agent, alcohol. I need hardly, indeed, presume to offer any suggestions, but one or two of a specially practical and every-day character may be ventured.

I am bound to intimate that the popular plan of administering alcohol for the purpose of sustaining the animal warmth is an entire and dangerous error, and that when it is brought into practice during extremely cold weather it is calculated to lead even to fatal consequences, from the readiness with which it permits the blood to become congested in the vital organs. I cannot too forcibly impress the fact that cold and alcohol act, physiologically, in the same manner, and that, combined in action, every danger resulting from either agent is doubled.

Whenever we see a person disposed to meet the effects of cold by strong drink it is our duty to endeavor to check that effort, and whenever we see an unfortunate person under the influence of alcohol it is our duty to suggest warmth as the best means for his recovery. These facts prompt many other useful ideas of detail, in our common life. If, for instance, our police were taught the simple art of taking the animal temperature of persons they have removed from the streets in a state of insensibility, the results would be most beneficial. The operation is one that hundreds of nurses now carry out daily, and applied by our police-officers, at their stations, it would enable them not only to suspect the difference between a man in an apoplectic fit and a man intoxicated, but would suggest naturally the instant abolition of the practice of thrusting the really intoxicated into a cold and damp cell, which to such a one is actually an anteroom to the grave.*

---

* Since the delivery of this lecture I am informed that in the London Metropolitan District the cells in which the intoxicated

Once more: I would earnestly impress that the systematic administration of alcohol for the purpose of giving and sustaining strength is an entire delusion. I am not going to say that occasions do not arise when an enfeebled or fainting heart is temporarily relieved by the relaxation of the vessels which alcohol, on its diffusion through the blood, induces; but that this spirit gives any persistent increase of power by which men are enabled to perform more sustained work is a mistake as serious as it is universal.

Again, the belief that alcohol may be used with advantage to fatten the body is, when it is acted upon, fraught with danger. For if we could successfully fatten the body we should but destroy it the more swiftly and surely; and as the fattening which follows the use of alcohol is not confined to the external development of fat but extends to a degeneration through the minute structures of the vital organs, including the heart itself, the danger is painfully apparent.

In conclusion, whatever good can come from alcohol, or whatever evil, is all included in that primary physiological and luxurious action of the agent upon the nervous supply of the circulation to which I have endeavored so earnestly to direct your attention. If it be really a luxury for the heart to be lifted up by alcohol; for the blood to course more swiftly through the brain; for the thoughts to flow more vehemently ; for words to

are received are not open to the objections named. I am glad to be able to make this correction.

come more fluently ; for emotions to rise ecstatically, and for life to rush on beyond the pace set by nature ; then those who enjoy the luxury must enjoy it,—with the consequences.

LECTURE V.

THE SECONDARY ACTION OF ALCOHOL ON THE ANIMAL FUNCTIONS, AND ON THE PHYSICAL DETERIORATIONS OF STRUCTURE INCIDENT TO ITS EXCESSIVE USE.

IT is my business in this course of lectures to treat upon the specific action of absolute alcohol. I have therefore specially avoided all reference to the spirituous drinks of which it forms a part. As a rule in every form of strong drink the source of the action of it, for good or for evil, is the spirit it contains, and the influence of the drink is potent according to the amount of that spirit present in it. To put the matter simply, if all the liquors sold under various names—wine, brandy, gin, rum, whisky, ale, stout, perry, cider,—were divested of their alcoholic spirit, they would contain comparatively little of anything that would affect those who partook of them.

DELETERIOUS ADDITIONS TO ALCOHOLIC DRINKS.

As I am, however, about to speak of the deleterious action of alcohol, it is fair I should admit that some bad effects do spring from so-called wine and kindred drinks independently of the pure spirit they contain. Something less of evil than now obtains would be secured if none but natural wines and ales were taken by the people. To return t ⟩ the times before brantwein was distilled, and to have no intoxicating beverages save pure wine and sound ale, were doubtless an improvement on the state of things which now exists; for, in truth, at the present time the characters of pure ethylic wine are hardly known. A *bonâ-fide* wine derived from the fermentation of the grape purely, cannot contain more than seventeen per cent. of alcohol, yet our staple wines, by an artificial process of fortifying and brandying, which means the adding of spirit, are brought up in sherries to twenty, and in ports to even twenty-five per cent. Some wines and spirits are believed to be charged with amylic alcohol. Other wines are charged with foreign volatile substances to impart what is called bouquet, and still other so-called wines—I allude specially to the effervescing liquids sold under that name—are actually often undergoing the fermenting process at the time they are imbibed, and thus are invited to complete their fermentation in that sensitive bottle, the human stomach.

If the subject were specially looked into, a very important chapter of facts might be collected bearing upon the injurious effects of these additions to ales, wines, and spirits. I have noticed the evils that follow upon the administration of an alcoholic drink that has been adulterated with amylic alcohol, and have shown that they are exceedingly serious. The disturbances excited by the other faults, when they do not arise from excess of absolute alcohol, are shown in symptoms of indigestion and in the promotion of an acid condition of the secretions of the body, beyond what is natural.

Presuming therefore it be actually determined by any one that he will take some alcoholic fluid, he will do nearest to that which is most wise if he takes wines or other spirituous drinks in which the quantity of alcohol is simply confined to the natural amount, in which the process of fermentation has ceased, and in which no foreign substance has been introduced to add either bouquet, body, piquancy, narcotising influence, or other artificial quality.

ABSINTHE.

The admitted addition of some actively poisonous substances to alcohol, in order to produce a new luxury, is the evil most disastrous. The drink sold under the name of *absinthe* is peculiarly formidable. In this liquor five drachms of the essence of absinthium, or wormwood, are added to one hundred quarts of alcohol. Thus the liquor is not only very strong as a mere alcoholic drink, but it is charged with another agent which has been discovered to exert the most powerful and dangerous action upon the nervous functions. The essence of absinthium in doses of from thirty to fifty grains produces in dogs and rabbits signs of extreme terror and trembling, followed by stupor and insensibility. In larger doses it causes epileptiform convulsions, foaming at the mouth, and stertor of the breathing. Its effects, as they occur from the taking of it in the form of absinthe in man, have been most ably described to me by one who indulged in it until it induced in him the peculiar epileptiform seizure. He described the effects as resembling those produced by *haschish*, the narcotic of the East which has been known for ages as the *nepenthes* of Homer, and which owes its properties to extract of Indian hemp or *Cannabis indica*. The partial insensibility caused by the absinthe is attended with the ideal existence of long intervals of time, in which the events of a whole life are arrayed and appreciated, to be succeeded by terrific hallucinations and intellectual weakness, ending in unconscious struggling as if for life. In time, if the use of the absinthe be continued, these phenomena become permanently established and the result is inevitably fatal.

The doubly poisonous absinthe is made the more seductive to its victims by the fact that it excites a morbid craving for food which is never felt except when it is tempted by the destroying agent. Indeed such are the terrible consequences incident to this agent, that I agree with Dr. Decaisne in maintaining that it ought, by legal provision, to be forbidden as an article for human consumption in all civilized communities. Even in small quantities taken daily, say one or two wineglassfuls, it causes quickly a permanent dyspepsia, and, what is of still more consequence, it tempts its victims on and on, so that they cannot take food until absinthe has prompted the desire for it, by which time they are too often hopelessly and mortally in its power.

Until recently absinthe has not been publicly offered for sale in this country on a large scale.

But now, unhappily, the poison is openly announced even here, and the consumption is on the increase ; I am doing therefore a public duty in denouncing its use solemnly from this platform, whence so much that is beneficial to society has for a century past been spoken.

ADDITION OF OTHER AGENTS.

The intentional additions of poisonous agents to the alcohol of ales, wines, and spirits pale when absinthe appears in sight, but they are not to be ignored. It is true that we very often hear accounts of the effects for evil of bad wine, when, in fact, the evil is due to the excess of ordinary alcohol that has been taken by the complainant. At the same time it is not to be denied that there exists in our midst a system of mixing, compounding, blending, and reducing wines and spirits, which, carried even to artistic perfection, is additionally prejudicial to the business of selling the various alcoholic beverages.

To be just to our own age, this artistic performance is not an invention of it. The adulteration of wine is indeed one of the oldest devices, extending from the Greeks and Romans onwards to this day. In the Middle Ages many prohibitory acts were passed against it by various governments. As late as the close of the seventeenth century an act was passed by Duke Everhard Louis of Würtemberg making it an offence punishable with death and confiscation of property to adulterate wine with bismuth, sulphur, or the salt of lead called litharge, now known as the yellow protoxide of lead. In the year 1705–6, John Jacob Ernhi, of Eslingen, was actually beheaded for carrying out adulteration with the forbidden poisonous lead compound.

Into our modern civilization a different system of treating strong drinks, in order to rectify bad qualities or to impart new, is, as a rule, followed. The plan of using gypsum or sulphate of lime to remove the acidity of wine, a practice that was followed both by the Greeks and Romans, is, however, still resorted to; so also is the practice of using lime for the same purpose, and for which Jack Falstaff so severely criticises the landlord of the " Boar's Head ":

" You rogue, here's lime in this sack: There is nothing but roguery to be found in villanous man: yet a coward is worse than a cup of sack with lime in it; a villanous coward."

But, on the whole, the new day has brought new plans and new intentions, having reference to the different forms of drinks, namely, ales, wines, and spirits, which pass from the hands of the vendor to the consumer.

ALES.

The practice of adulteration the least hurtful is carried on in ales; that at all events is my experience of the ales sold in London, and I speak from a practical knowledge of the facts. A few years ago a well-known statist asked me to undertake for him a research on the ales sold in London, with a view to the detection of the adulterations in them. For many weeks this gentleman himself

collected beers and ales from different retail houses
in the most diverse parts of this metropolis, and
neither trouble nor expense was spared in the examination of these samples, in order to arrive at
correct results as to the composition of the fluids
thus retailed. I may state at once that I did not
in any one instance find a truly dangerous adulteration. I found that to many samples common salt
had been added, and to some sugar; but the grand
adulteration was water, by which the consumer
was, if I may so express it, fraudulently benefited
and the government proportionately defrauded. If
this aqueous adulteration were not carried on, our
registrars of deaths and collectors of revenues
would both show heavier totals.

There is a prevailing notion that to malt liquor,
bitter substances, such as strychnine, or narcotic
substances, such as *cocculus indicus*, are added.
Neumann says that in his time, that is just one
hundred years ago, *clary*, *cocculus indicus*, and
Bohemian rosemary were added to malt liquors in
order to increase their intoxicating powers, and he
states that the last-named substance, Bohemian
rosemary, produced a raving intoxication. I know
it is also urged, in this day, that there is no known
application for the quantity of *cocculus indicus* that
is sold except it be for the adulteration of malt
liquors. I will not dispute the matter, but I content myself with stating that I have never detected
any foreign body of the kind, and that in the whole
of my experience of the effect of malt liquors on
man, I have never known a symptom produced
indicative of the effects of such substances.

The stronger ales and stouts are injurious mainly from the alcohol they contain. Those which
have not ceased fermenting, and from which
gas is escaping, produce a persistent dyspepsia
in persons who indulge in them, a dyspepsia attended with flatulency, painful distension of the
stomach, and with loss of proper muscular power
of the stomach, by which deficiency the trituration
of food is impeded and rendered imperfect. At
the same time the action of the gastric fluids upon
the food is made less effective. There is at the
present day in the market a substance used as an
addition to ales, which is called *saccharina*. It is
sold in the form of the ordinary sugar-loaf. It is
made by the action of diluted sulphuric acid upon
starchy matter, and is, in fact, a grape sugar. It
gives to the ale body and sweetness. It is in itself
a fattening food, and as it is the same as that form
of sugar which is found in those who suffer from
the disease called diabetes, and which produces the
symptoms of that disease, it cannot be taken in
quantity without some indirect risk of danger.

WINES.

The evils arising from wines, apart from those
which are due to the natural ethylic alcohol they
should contain, are derived from several sources.
The wine that has not ceased to ferment, and when
uncorked is found to be charged with gas, is often
as injurious as beer in which the fermentation has
not ended. It produces a fermenting process
within the body, and gives rise to those phenomena of dyspepsia to which allusion has already been

made. Wine that has once been acid and has been
treated with lime in order that the acidity may be
neutralised, is open to the objection of an excess
of salts of lime. It has been urged against wines
treated in this manner that they lead to calculous
disease when they are taken in quantity for long
periods. I must answer to this suggestion that I
have not had experience of the slightest evidence
that would support it, nor do I think there is sufficient of such wine consumed to warrant any conclusion of the kind. Wine if adulterated with
amylic alcohol is unquestionably dangerous, owing
to those physiological effects produced by the
adulterant to which I specially directed attention
in the second lecture of this course. Wines that
are beaded are injurious, owing to the foreign
mixture for beading that has been added to them,
and which I shall presently describe.

Some substances that form in natural wines exert an effect on the animal body when they are
taken into it. These substances are principally
aldehyde and acetic acid. Aldehyde when it is
present in wine communicates to it a natural bouquet. You will find on the table a pure specimen
of aldehyde, and you will also find specimens of
natural wines, kindly lent to me by Mr. Denman,
in which this change of alcohol by oxidation has
taken place. In the year 1848 the late Sir James
Simpson, of Edinburgh, discovered that aldehyde
would produce anæsthetic sleep when its vapor
was inhaled, and I have since submitted it to experiment with a view of testing its action on the
living body. I find it is a rapidly intoxicating

agent, sharp to the nerves of sense, and acting
with greater rapidity than alcohol, and with a less
prolonged effect, for it is soluble in water, and is
so volatile that it boils at 72° Fahr.   It is therefore quickly diffused and quickly eliminated from
the body.   The action of aldehyde upon the living body has been as yet insufficiently studied.
It has a close relation to the narcotic action of alcohol, and the symptoms it produces are so similar
I am inclined to believe that the narcotism which
follows the administration of alcoholic spirit is
partly due to its production.

The presence of acetic acid in wines is on the
whole not injurious, if the wine in other respects
be free of adulteration.   The tendency of this acid
itself is to promote the digestion of albuminous
foods, and I have sometimes observed in persons
whose digestive power is feeble, signs of improvement under its use.   In saying this I do not however wish to convey that therefore a rough acid
wine should be taken for indigestion, for the acid
in such instances may be administered without the
wine and perhaps with greater advantage.   I only
wish to record that acidity of wine, in which fermentation has ceased, is not a source of additional
injury.   The astringent acid—called tannic—of
some wines has been advanced as useful in the
cases of certain persons who suffer from laxity of
body, and who require astringent remedies.   It
would be wrong to dispute that there may be in
wine a virtue of this kind, but it is not peculiar
to wine.   It can be secured when it is wanted
without wine at all, and in a more certain way.

This remark holds equally good in respect to what may be favorably spoken of as the saline substances which some wines naturally present. I mean to say that the saline constituents can be administered with more certain and therefore with better effect, independently of wine.

SPIRITS.

Into the different spirits commonly sold, several substances are introduced which exert more or less of baneful influence on the body that receives them. The addition of amylic alcohol has been already condemned and need not again be mentioned, and I omit intentionally, for the sake of brevity, a great number of other added substances which do not seem to me to be active for evil, though they were possibly better left out of the animal organism. After these are withdrawn there remain many other agents which cannot fairly be omitted from our consideration. There is oil of juniper, oil of bitter almonds, potassa, alum, nitric acid, oil of vitriol, or sulphuric acid, and butyric acid. In even small quantities every one of these agents is injurious to the body if it be taken for any long continued period of time. The oil of juniper is an active diuretic, and thereby is injurious to the excreting power of one of the most important of the vital organs. The oil of bitter almonds contains, unless it be specially purified, hydrocyanic or prussic acid, and exerts then in small and often-repeated quantities a prejudicial influence on the nervous functions. Potassa causes a dry and caustic action upon the mucous membrane of the mouth, throat, and stomach, for the production of which action it is actually added systematically, that it may give the peculiar sharpness called " biting the palate."

Alum is a powerful astringent, producing constipation, and sustaining a persistent dyspepsia so long as it is being swallowed. Nitric acid is an astringent, exerting also a physiological action on the liver. Sulphuric acid is an astringent; and butyric acid, as I found in an original research which I once conducted with it, causes a congested or inflammatory condition of the whole track of the mucous membrane.

Thus each one of these agents added to the alcoholic drinks increases the evils that are likely to arise from the alcohol itself. Let us admit that the added evils are small, nay, I had nearly said, infinitesimal, when considered by the measurement of one administration. But who can measure by that standard? When once the taste for any of these unnatural substances is acquired it grows by what it feeds on, and that which was infinitesimal at the beginning becomes after long continuance a serious charge for the body to bear daily.

The spirit in common use that is most subject to the chemicals I have named is gin. Gin has to be made cordial, to be sweetened, to be rendered creamy and smooth, to be flavored, to be made biting to the palate, to be beaded, and what not else. To be made "cordial" it must be charged with oil of juniper, with essence of angelica, with oil of bitter almonds, with oil of coriander, and with oil of carraway. To sweeten it, it must be treated with oil of vitriol, oil of almonds, oil of juniper, spirits of wine and loaf sugar; to "force down" the same it must be further treated with a solution of alum and carbonate of potassa. To be rendered creamy and smooth, it must be sweetened with sugar, and lightly charged with a small quantity of garlic, Canadian balsam, or Strasburg turpentine. To give it piquancy, it must have had digested in it shreds of horse-radish. To be made biting to the palate, it must receive that touch of caustic potash of which I have spoken.

As you see the habituated gin-drinker partaking of his favorite drink you observe, often, that he enjoys it the more if it be what he calls "pearly," or "beaded." He holds up the precious liquid in his glass, and as he sees the oily fluid roll down the side, as beads, leaving each a creamy train behind it, he rejoices in his treasure. It is *crême de la crême* of gin. Those wicked, pearly drops are, to his flushed eyes, the proofs of the purity and excellence of what he would probably tell you was, without mistake, the genuine article. The genuineness consists in the fact that our enthusiastic friend's gin has been beaded by the addition of the following artistic mixture :—An ounce of oil of sweet almonds has been added to an ounce of oil of vitriol. These have been rubbed together in a mortar with two ounces of loaf sugar until a paste has been formed. The paste has next been dissolved in spirit of wine until a thin liquid has been produced; and this, added to one hundred gallons of gin, has given the fine pearly bead that is so much admired.

Redding, in his history and description of modern wines, narrated in his day the many receipts that were openly published in the then existing publicans' guides and licensed victuallers' directories for the artificial manufacturing of wines, and for modifying spirituous liquors. I have gone for my information to a similar work of the present day, "The New Mixing and Reducing Book," which is, I understand, one of the handbooks of the retailer, the same to him as the pharmacopœia is to the druggist, and to be followed in all the varied arts as implicitly. I cannot leave this book without reading from it a quotation that bears directly on the health of the poorer classes, who indulge in gin.

"Gin, it may be observed, is of all the spirits ordinarily kept by a publican the one which, when cleverly managed, yields him the greatest and securest profit. The reason of this is that there is hardly any definite selling strength for gin, especially if it be sweetened. Within very wide limits no complaint is made by customers on the score of weakness, provided only the gin is creamy, palatable, and sharp tasted. But the slightest taint, or the slightest fault of color, or a sensible difference in the usual flavor, will lead to dissatisfaction and loss of custom. Strong or unsweetened gin is in comparatively little request, and then with few exceptions only amongst the respectable or monied classes. At least three-fourths of the spirits sold over the counter of a public house consists of a sweetened or made-up gin; and as the sugar greatly alters the character of the liquor and deadens the original strength, it is possible for the retailer to consult his own interests by a liberal addition of water without in any degree exciting the disapprobation, or injuring the health of those who patronise his establishment.

"As a tolerably safe general rule there will be no occasion to fear dissatisfaction when sweetened gin is not brought below 35 or even 40 per cent. U. P. It is then nearly five times as strong as old ale. Much more is thought of a pleasant warming aromatic taste or smack than of simple alcoholic strength. But as the most careful man may sometimes overshoot the mark in reducing, it is advisable to know how to restore the requisite degree of pungency and sharpness, without having recourse to the use of so expensive an agent as spirit of wine. Supposing, then, that by accident the strength of a parcel of gin has been lowered rather too far, a good and cheap remedy is the following : —For 100 gallons, 1 ounce of cassia, ½ ounce of chilies. Steep for a week in a pint of spirit of wine ; then mix well with the gin."

The other spirituous liquors, rum, whisky, and brandy, are less falsified than gin. Rum is occasionally adulterated with an essential oil like butyrin and with butyric acid, these two substances being present in some natural rum, to which they give a special flavor. Whisky is modified by blending, so as to communicate qualities of smoothness and softness. The yellowish color given to whisky is produced by pouring the spirit into sherry casks, or by stirring it up with the lees of wine. These refined whiskies are prepared for the rich and sumptuous ; the poor, it is recommended, should be treated with the spirit they understand best ; a sharp and potent drink, that will bring the tears into the eyes, and make the throat smart as it goes down.

Brandy, except when treated with fusel oil, is not, I believe, adulterated with any injurious compound. But it carries with it naturally a peculiar ether, which gives to it a special odor. This ether is very heavy when compared with ethylic ether. Its specific gravity is 862, taking water at 1,000, and its boiling point is 479° on Fahrenheit's scale. It is all but insoluble in water, to which, however, it communicates its peculiar odor. It exerts on the body an injurious influence ; it causes nausea, thirst, and pain in the stomach. It seems also to arrest the due secretion of bile.

SECONDARY PHYSIOLOGICAL ACTION OF SIMPLE ALCOHOL.

I leave now the consideration of the evils arising from the action of the different extraneous substances that are present in alcoholic drinks to resume the study of the action of ethylic alcohol itself when it is free of any such combinations. I have to consider under this head the effect of the consumption of alcohol in its slow and progressive course, in what may be called its secondary manifestations of effect upon those who for long periods of their lives submit themselves to its influence.

I have shown that in the course of acute intoxication from this spirit there are four degrees or stages, each degree marked by different series of phenomena. In the secondary, or, technically speaking, chronic intoxication, from the same agent, there are in like manner four distinct degrees, each presenting distinct phenomena. A minority of persons who habitually take alcohol escape with impunity from injury. Some of these escape because they only subject themselves to it on a scale so moderate they can scarcely be said to be under its spell. If they take it regularly they never exceed an ounce to an ounce and a half of the pure spirit in the day; and if they indulge in a little more than this, it is only at recreative seasons, after which they atone for what they have done by a temporary total abstinence. Others take more freely than the above, but escape because they are physiologically constituted in such manner that they can rapidly eliminate the fluid from their bodies. These, if they are moderately prudent, may even go so far as to indulge in alcohol and yet suffer no material harm. But they are a limited few, if the term may be applied to them, who are thus privileged. The large majority of those who drink alcohol in any of its disguises are injured by it. As a cause of disease it gives origin to great populations of afflicted persons, many of whom suffer even to death without suspecting from what they suffer, and unsuspected. Some of these live just short of the first stage of natural old age; others to ripe middle age; others only to ripe adolescence.

DETERIORATION OF THE BODY UNDER THE FIRST
DEGREE.

The first degree of the secondary action of alcohol is evidenced in those who by constant habit
imbibe an alcoholic stimulant to the simple extent
of producing arterial relaxation, and of setting the
heart at liberty to perform an increased series of
motive contractions. They do not, as a rule, receive what is commonly called an excess of any alcoholic drink, but they become trained to a sensation of want for it and to an appetite which, while
all seems to go well, they have no desire to resist,
though they may keep it within what they conceive
are its due limits. Such persons confine their liba-
tions to four or six ounces of alcohol per day, a
couple of glasses of sherry or of ale at luncheon,
three or four glasses of wine at dinner, one or two
at dessert, and a mixture of spirit and water before
going to bed. Such is a common and a " temperate day," but reckoned up it means at least from
four to six ounces of alcohol. The primary effect
of such a quantity we know. Continued daily it
induces a new physiological and altogether unnatural condition, in which the sense of acquired necessity enforces desire, until at last the spirit is
made to became a positive requirement of the organic and the mental life. Every extra effort must
be preceded by the resort to the stimulant. Every
prolonged weariness must be relieved by the same
measure; but when the effect of the stimulant has
speedily subsided, there is left a greater exhaustion
than before. Another resource to the artificial aid

completes the exhaustion, and makes it pass into dulness and drowsiness without natural and sound sleep, and with an unbearable sense of after prostration.

For many years, in the young and adolescent, this alcoholic life may be carried on without any evidence being rendered of the progress of physical deterioration. In the young the processes of assimilation, of secretion, and of excretion, are in their full activity, and the poisonous agent with which the blood and tissues are saturated is disposed of so readily and promptly, it does not stay long enough in contact with these parts to vitiate them. This is a very homely way of putting the fact, but it is scientifically true. The young, therefore, seem to escape, and I believe that up to the close of the first term of the natural life, that is to say, to the close of that period of full growth and development which extends to thirty years, they sometimes escape so successfully that if they could but stop in their course at that point they might go through the remaining terms of existence without any further important modification of function.

Unfortunately, it is the rarest of events that a person artificially stimulated by alcohol, to the period named, gives up the practice. The majority are utterly ignorant of the dangers that are ahead, and the sense of support to which they have been educated by the practice leads them on to pursue it with even a greater reliance upon it than before, and with a feeling of more urgent demand. In a word, the sensation that they cannot do without it, the sensation of lowness and depression when it is by any accident withheld, and the contrast of lightness and activity when it is regained, are so powerful, in their influences upon the mind, there is no resisting the belief of the absolute necessity.

But when the body is fully developed; when the extra vital capacity which attended youth is expended in growth and development; when all the organs have assumed their full size and activity; when the balance of secretion is so nicely set in all parts that not one secretion can be disturbed without a disturbance of the whole; when the spring of the elastic tissues is reduced; when the lungs cannot fail ever so little in their function of throwing off the gaseous products of combustion without a vicarious extrusion of gases into the alimentary canal; when the completed organic moving parts become encumbered with fatty matter interposed between them, or laid out around them; then the effect of alcoholic spirits begins to be realised. The fluid is now retained longer in the living house; is decomposed less quickly; is thrown out by primary or secondary elimination less speedily.

The action of alcohol under these new conditions, so favorable in every sense to the series of changes it is capable of effecting, is twofold. The action in the first place is purely mechanical. We are aware that it leads to temporary paralysis of the vessels of the minute circulation, and that upon this the heart responds with a quicker propelling stroke. Thus the vessels throughout the whole of the body are dilated, and are held in a state of unnatural relaxation and unnatural tension. Under this persistent pressure their diameters change in course of time, and the whole of the marvellous webwork of blood, upon which the organs of the body are constructed, is deranged, in its mechanical distribution, over its extended surface. During this time, too, the function of the heart becomes perverted. The heart is truly an automatic organ, but it is still an organ which feels none the less severely the effect of the stimulus. If it make to-day an unnatural number of one hundred and twenty-five thousand strokes, it cannot to-morrow sink back, from absence of its stimulus, to the normal one hundred thousand without evidencing some disturbance of action, some feebleness, some hesitation, or some palpitation. In fact, as it is an organ which by its own stroke feeds its own structure with blood, it is the first to suffer from irregular supplies of blood. Thus, under alcohol, the nutrition of the heart is mechanically modified. Whipped into undue work, it becomes like the muscles of the blacksmith's arm or the opera-dancer's leg, of undue size and power; and in proportion as this evil increases, the necessity for the stimulus it calls for grows more urgent.

In turn this extreme power and force of the heart tells upon the vessels that are fed by its impulsive stroke, and so all the organs that are constructed upon those vessels appreciate with abnormal sensitiveness the whip of the stimulus, and the languor when the whip is withheld.

Of itself this extreme sensitiveness of the heart is sufficiently momentous, but the ultimate results upon the body at large are perhaps more important than the pure local change that is instituted in that perfect and elaborate pulsating mechanism. The heart not only becomes enlarged, but its various valvular and other mechanical parts, subjected to prolonged strain, are thrown out of proportion. The orifices in it, through which the great floods of blood issue in their courses, are dilated. The exquisite valves become stretched, and prevented from assuming their refined adaptations. The minute filamentous cords which hold the valves in due position and tension are elongated, and the walls of the ventricles or forcing-chambers are thickened, or as we say, technically, are hypertrophied. Throughout the whole of its structures the central throbbing organ is modified both in its mechanism and in its action.

But such central modification cannot possibly go on long without the institution of other changes at the opposite extremity or circumference of the circuit of the blood. At one moment the vital organs feel the pressure of the too powerful stroke of blood; at another moment they are suddenly aware of an enfeebled stroke. The brain is, for the instant, conscious of a flicker of power: it is like the faintest flicker of gas, which is observed when, by an accident, the pressure is disturbed at the main, but it is there, and the person who experiences it is cognisant of its central origin. So matters progress often for months, or for years, without further evidence of subjective or objective sign of increasing evil. The worst evidence that exists is, probably, the necessity for a more frequent repetition of the stimulus under additional stress of work or excitement.

While these changes in the simple mechanism of the circulation are in course of advancement, there are also in development certain other changes which are much more delicate and minute, yet not less important. These consist of direct deteriorations of structure of the organic tissues themselves. We are, at the present time, only on the border-land of a new knowledge on this subject, and I myself am, in this matter, a mere outpost wandering wonderingly, and trying to observe what is going on, but as yet, though thus advanced, unprepared to speak with so much precision and fulness of detail as I would desire. The following explanation, simply spoken, illustrates the degenerative changes of organic structure from the continued use of alcohol.

Alcohol produces physical deterioration by destroying the integrity of the colloidal matter of which the tissues are composed. I have explained that all the organic parts are constructed out of colloidal substance ; that every such part, including the blood-vessels, to their minutest ramifications, is composed of this colloid material arranged in different forms and plans to suit the design of the part, whether it be a tube, like an artery, a bundle of cross-cut fibres like a muscle, or a refracting globe like the crystalline lens of the eyeball. That these parts should be kept in their integrity, in the midst of their diversity, the ultimate structure of which they are composed must be held in proper measure of construction with water. Disturb the relationship that should exist between the colloid and its combining water, and the character of the colloid is at once changed. Take, for example, some colloidal albumen in the fluid state. Pour a little of it on to a glass plate as a thin watery film. Then spread over it a little finely powdered caustic soda, by which to remove and fix some of the water which previously held it as a liquid. The thin liquid is transformed into a transparent membrane which possesses elasticity. Into a porcelain cup pour a small quantity of the same solution, and then drop into the solution a bead of soda; soon you can lift the solution from the cup in a solid mass, shaped like a concavo-convex transparent lens. I could multiply these facts indefinitely, but I am anxious to indicate only one particular fact, viz., that alcohol and its derivative aldehyde possess also, by their affinity for water, the property of destroying the integrity of the colloidal form of matter. Thus they solidify, or render pectous the colloidal structures. Take a solution of albumen and add to it alcohol. The albumen is rendered thick or pectous. Take a solution of caseine; add to it aldehyde; the caseine is rendered thick or pectous.

Animal tissues subjected to alcohol can be perverted to any degree, and in the most diverse and apparently contradictory ways. I can hold blood permanently fluid with alcohol; I can solidify it with the same agent. I can reduce the size and modify the shape of the blood corpuscles, and I can so modify those fine and delicate animal membranes which dialyse or allow to pass through them the saline matter of the blood and secretions, that the process of dialysis shall be impeded, and that which should pass through shall be left in combination with the membrane. I can destroy the elasticity of the blood-vessels in the same way, for that depends upon the presence in them of a gelatinous colloid elasticity also called elasticin.

When, therefore, alcohol holds long-continued contact with the perfectly developed colloidal tissues, its action upon them to produce physical deterioration is simply inevitable, and from this cause arise those fatal lesions of local organs which mark the different phases and stages of alcoholic disease. The commencement of the change sometimes shows itself visibly on the surface of the body. The vessels of the face become permanently enlarged and suffused with blood. In cold weather, the blood circulating imperfectly through these vessels, and, not fully aërated, gives to the skin that dull leaden hue which is so characteristically significant of prolonged indulgence. In hot weather, the blood circulating more freely and purely, gives to. the skin a red hue and often a deep red blotch, which is hardly less demonstrative.

In this stage of alcoholic disease eruptions upon the skin occur to declare the injurious action of the spirit upon the colloidal gelatinous textures. The epidermis or scarf-skin is imperfectly thrown off; it dies upon the surface, but owing to deficient vascular and nervous tone beneath, it is not replaced so quickly as is natural. Thus the dead *débris*, in form of scale and sometimes with fluid beneath, accumulates; the superficial nervous surface which should be protected by the newly formed epidermis is exposed, and irritation and pain follow as a consequence.

The evils, in the slighter stages of alcoholic disease, are often connected with others, which are perhaps passing, but which give rise to very unpleasant phenomena. There is what is called a dyspepsia or indigestion, to relieve which the sufferer too frequently resorts to the actual cause of it as the cure for it. There is thirst, there is uneasiness of the stomach, flatulency, and a set of so-called nervous phenomena, which keep the mind irritable, and make trifling cares and anxieties assume an exaggerated and unnatural character. From the earliest period in the history of the drinking of alcohol these phenomena have been observed. "Who," says Solomon, referring to this action, "Who hath woe? Who hath contentions? Who hath babbling? Who hath wounds without cause? Who hath redness of the eyes?"

What modern physiologist could define better the steady and progressive effect of alcohol upon those who, even under the guise of temperate men, trust to it as a support? And yet these evils are minor compared with certain I have to bring forward in the next and concluding lecture.

LECTURE VI.

PHYSICAL DETERIORATIONS FROM ALCOHOL (*continued*).—INFLUENCE OF ALCOHOL ON THE VITAL ORGANS.—MENTAL PHENOMENA INDUCED BY ITS USE.—SUMMARY.

TOWARDS the close of my last lecture I touched on the effects of the continued action of alcohol upon the colloidal structures of the body, indicating that it is impossible for these structures to escape deterioration. I must dwell for a few moments longer on this subject.

The parts which first suffer most from alcohol are those expansions in the animal body which the anatomists call the membranes. The membranes are colloidal structures, and every organ is enveloped in them. The skin is a membranous envelope. Through the whole of the alimentary surface, from the lips downwards, and through the bronchial passages to their minutest ramifications, extends the mucous membrane. The lungs, the heart, the liver, the kidneys are folded in delicate membranes which can be stripped easily from these parts. If you take a portion of bone, you will find it easy to strip off from it a membranous sheath or covering; if you open and examine a joint you will find both the head and the socket lined with membrane.

149

The whole of the intestines are enveloped in fine membrane called *peritoneum*. All the muscles are enveloped in membranes, and the fasciculi or bundles and fibres of muscles have their membranous sheathing. The brain and spinal cord are enveloped in three membranes; one nearest to themselves, a pure vascular structure, a net-work of blood-vessels; another, a thin serous structure; a third, a strong fibrous structure. The eyeball is a structure of colloidal humors and membranes, and of nothing else. To complete the description, the minute structures of the vital organs are enrolled in membranous matter.

It was held by the old anatomists that this membranous arrangement of the body is mainly mechanical. The parts and organs, according to their · view, are supported and held in position by these membranous sheaths and pouches and coverings. Doubtless this is a portion of their usefulness, for in fact they do hold all the structures together in the most perfect order. But this is only a small part of their duties. The membranes are the filters of the body. In their absence there could be no building of structure, no solidification of tissue, no organic mechanism. Passive themselves, they nevertheless separate all structures into their respective positions and adaptations.

The animal receives from the vegetable world and from the earth the food and drink it requires for its sustenance and motion. It receives colloidal food for its muscles; combustible food for its motion; water for the solution of its various parts; salt for constructive and other physical purposes.

These have all to be arranged in the body ; and they are arranged by means of the membranous envelopes. Through these membranes nothing can pass that is not for the time in a state of aqueous solution like water or soluble salts. Water passes freely through them, salts pass freely through them, but the constructive matter of the active parts that is colloidal does not pass ; it is retained in them until it is chemically decomposed into the soluble type of matter. When we take for our food a portion of animal flesh, it is first resolved, in digestion, into a soluble fluid before it can be absorbed ; in the blood it is resolved into the fluid colloidal condition ; in the solids it is laid down within the membranes into new structure, and when it has played its part it is digested again, if I may so say, into a crystalloidal soluble substance ready to be carried away and replaced by addition of new matter, then it is dialysed or passed through the membranes into the blood, and is disposed of in the excretions.

See then what an all-important part these membranous structures play in the animal life. Upon their integrity all the silent work of the building up of the body depends. If these membranes are rendered too porous, and let out the colloidal fluids of the blood—the albumen for example—the body so circumstanced dies ; dies as if it were slowly bled to death. If, on the contrary, they become condensed or thickened, or loaded with foreign material, then they fail to allow the natural fluids to pass through them. They fail to dialyse, and the result is, either an accumulation of the fluid in a closed cavity, or contraction of the substance enclosed within the membrane, or dryness of membrane in surfaces that ought to be freely lubricated and kept apart. In old age we see the effects of modification of membrane naturally induced; we see the fixed joint, the shrunken and feeble muscle, the dimmed eye, the deaf ear, the enfeebled nervous function.

It may possibly seem at first sight that I am leading immediately away from the subject of the secondary action of alcohol. It is not so. I am leading directly to it. Upon all these membranous structures alcohol exerts a direct perversion of action. It produces in them a thickening, a shrinking, and an inactivity that reduces their functional power. That they may work rapidly and equally they require to be at all times charged with water to saturation. If into contact with them any agent is brought that deprives them of water, then is their work interfered with; they cease to separate the saline constituents properly, and, if the evil that is thus started be allowed to continue, they contract upon their contained matter in whatever organ it may be situated, and condense it.

In brief, under the prolonged influence of alcohol those changes which take place from it in the blood corpuscles, and which have already been described, extend to the other organic parts, involving them in structural deteriorations, which are always dangerous, and are often ultimately fatal.

PRIMARY EFFECTS ON VITAL FUNCTIONS.

I remarked in my last lecture that the slow or

chronic effect of alcoholic drink upon the body was to induce a series of stages analogous in all respects, except in period of duration, to the process of acute poisoning by the same agent. In the first prolonged stage there occur phenomena of disease which are as characteristic of the agency, when it is known, as they are deceptive when the agency is not known.

The ultimate changes that follow the use of alcohol by those who indulge in it, in what is too often considered a temperate degree, are actual local changes within one or other of the vital organs. But before such actual deterioration obtains there are usually other phenomena transitory in character yet unequivocal. I pointed out certain of these in the last lecture, but I did not specify them all.

In addition to that irritation of mind and suffering " of wounds without cause," to which I then drew attention, an extreme emotional derangement is often produced. The afflicted man—and I fear I must say woman also, for women are sometimes afflicted—the afflicted man under this primary prolonged influence of alcohol becomes nervous and excitable, ready at any moment to cry or to laugh, without valid reasons for either act. The emotional centres are alternately raised and depressed in function by the poison, but after a time the depression overcomes the exhilaration, and the impulse is to a maudlin sentimentality extending even to tears. The slightest anxieties are then exaggerated, and there is experienced at the same time an indecision and deficiency of self-confidence which is doubly perplexing. When an act is done,

when a letter, for instance, or other piece of business
has been finished and despatched, an uneasy feeling
of distrust is felt that perhaps some mistake has
been made, which distrust passes rapidly into a
sentiment that the thing cannot be helped; it is
bad luck, but it must take its chance. In various
other directions this distrust shows itself, and the
worst of all is, that the very doubt prompts the
desire for another application for relief to the evil
that is the cause of the burthen. A small dram
more of the stimulant, not an overpowering draught
that will cause quick and sure insensibility, but just
a mouthful, that is the assumed remedy, and that
is the certain promoter of the sorrow.

We know now, as surely as if we could see within the body, what is the condition of the organs of
the person afflicted in the manner thus defined.
We are conscious that the vessels of the brain, of
the lungs, of the liver, of the kidneys, of the stomach
are paralysed, and are injected to full distention
with blood. Some of these parts have actually
been seen under this state, and the fact of the red
injected condition directly demonstrated.

Alcoholic Dyspepsia.

Of all the systems of organs that suffer under
this sustained excitement and paralysis, two are
injured most determinately, viz., the digestive and
the nervous. The stomach, unable to produce in
proper quantity the natural digestive fluid, and
also unable to absorb the food which it may imperfectly digest, is in constant anxiety and irritation. It is oppressed with the sense of nausea; it

is oppressed with the sense of emptiness and prostration ; it is oppressed with a sense of distention ;
it is oppressed with a loathing for food, and it is
teased with a craving for more drink. Thus there
is engendered a permanent disorder which, for
politeness' sake, is called dyspepsia, and for which
different remedies are often sought but never found.
Antibilious pills—whatever they may mean—Seid-
litz powders, effervescing waters, and all that pharmacopœia of aids to further indigestion, in which
the afflicted who nurse their own diseases so liber-
ally and innocently indulge, are tried in vain. I do
not strain a syllable when I state that the worst
forms of confirmed indigestion originate in the
practice that is here explained. By this practice
all the functions are vitiated, the skin at one moment is flushed and perspiring, at the next is pale,
cold, and clammy, and every other secreting structure is equally disarranged.

Nervous Derangements.

The nervous structures follow, or it may be pre-
cede, the stomach in the order of derangement.
We have not yet traced out with sufficient care
the conditions of the centres of the organic chain
of nerves, but we know that they are reduced in
power ; and, in regard to those higher and reasoning centres, the brain and its subsidiary parts, the
spinal cord and voluntary nerves, we are aware
that they are supplied with blood through vessels
weakened, and in a condition either of undue tension or undue relaxation. Moreover, the delicate
membranes which envelope and immediately sur-

round the nervous cords are acted upon more readily by the alcohol than the coarser membranous textures of other parts, and thus a combined arrangement of evils affects the nervous matter. The perverted condition of the nervous centres gives rise to many striking phenomena, extending from them to the nervous cords and to the organs of sense. The irregular supply of blood to the retina causes temporary disturbances of vision, with appearances before the eyes of those specks and small rounded semi-transparent discs, which are called by the learned *muscæ volitantes*. From the imperfect tension of the arteries, the blood which rushes through them causes their dilatation, and in the bony canals of the skull an impingement is made upon the bony structure. Vibrations which extend to the neighboring organs of hearing are thus produced, giving rise to sounds of a murmuring, ringing, or humming character, according to the modification of the arterial tension.

The perverted condition of the membranous covering of the nerves gives rise to pressure within the sheath of the nerve, and to pain as a consequence. To the pain thus excited the term neuralgia is commonly applied, or tic ; or if the large nerve running down the thigh be the seat of the pain, "sciatica." Sometimes this pain is developed as a tooth-ache. It is pain commencing in nearly every instance at some point where a nerve is enclosed in a bony cavity, or where pressure is easily excited, as at the lower jawbone near the centre of the chin, or at the opening in front of the lower part of the ear, or at the opening over the eyeball in the frontal bone.

Alcoholic Insomnia or Sleeplessness.

Lastly on this head, the perverted state of the vessels of the brain itself, the unnatural tension to which they are subjected from the stroke of the heart they are now so incompetent to resist, sets up in the end one telling, and of all I have yet named, most serious phenomenon ; I mean *insomnia* —inability to partake of natural sleep. There is a theory held by some physiologists that sleep is induced by the natural contraction of the minute vessels of the brain, and by the extrusion, through that contraction, of the blood from the brain. I am myself inclined, for reasons I need not wait to specify now, to consider this theory incorrect; but it is nevertheless true that during natural sleep the brain is receiving a reduced supply of blood ; that when the vessels are filled with blood without extreme distention, the brain remains awake, and that when the vessels are engorged and over-distended, there is induced an insensibility which is not natural sleep, but which partakes of the nature of apoplexy. This sleep is attended with long and embarrassed breathing, blowing expirations, deep snoring inspirations, and uneasy movements of the body, even with convulsive motions. From such sleep the apparent sleeper awakes unrefreshed and unready for the labors of the day. The effect of alcohol then on the brain is to maintain the relaxation of vessels, to keep the brain

charged with blood, and so to hold back the natural repose.   Under this form of divergence from
the natural life, the sleepless man lies struggling
with unruly and unconnected trains of thought.
He tries to force sleep by suppressing with a great
effort all thought, but in an instant wakes again.
At last the more he tries the less he succeeds, until
the morning dawns.   By that long time the spirit
that kept his cerebral vessels disabled and his
heart in wild unrest having become eliminated, he
is set free, and the coveted sleep follows.   Or perhaps, wearied of waiting for the normal results, he
rises, and with an additional dose of the great dis-
turber, or with some other tempting narcotic drug
of kindred nature, such as chloral, he so intensifies
the vascular paralysis as to plunge himself into the
oblivion of congestion, with those attendant apoplectic phenomena, which he himself hears not,
but which, to those who do hear, are alarming
in what they forebode, when their full meaning is
appreciated.   Connected with this sleep there is
engendered in some persons a form of true epilepsy, which all the skill of physic is hopeless to
cure, until the cause is revealed and removed.

And now I think I have said everything that I
have time to say respecting the general phenomena incident to this primary stage of slow
alcoholic intoxication in those who, in the world's
eye, as well as in their own, are temperate individuals—individuals who enjoy the choice things
of this life heartily ; who understand a glass of
wine, and who can take a good many glasses—or
a good many little "goes" of spirit if that be all

—but who are never known by friend or foe to be worse for anything they take; who grow mellow as an apple under the mellowing cheer, but never fall, nor lose their power of taking less guarded companions safely home.

ORGANIC DETERIORATIONS.

The continuance of the effects of alcohol into a more advanced stage leads to direct disorganisation of vital structures. When once this stage has been reached not one organ of the body escapes the ravage. According to the build or the hereditary construction of the individual, however, or according sometimes to what may be considered as a local accident, some particular organ undergoes a change which gives a specific character to the whole of the phenomena that are afterwards presented. We then say of the person in whom such change occurs that he is afflicted with such a particular disease, letting the general sink into the local manifestation. Many purely local modifications of structures and parts are in this manner induced in the blood, in the minute structure of the moving organs—the muscles, in the fixed vital organs, such as the brain, the lungs, the liver, the heart, the kidneys. In the blood the influence is exerted upon the plastic fibrine and upon the corpuscles; in the brain, on the membranes at first, and afterwards on the nervous matter they enclose; in the lungs, on the elastic, spongy, connective tissue, which is, strictly speaking, also membranous; in the heart, on its muscular elements and membranes; in the liver, primarily on its membranes;

in the kidneys, on their connective tissues and membranes.

SPECIAL STRUCTURAL DETERIORATIONS.

The organ of the body that perhaps the most frequently undergoes structural changes from alcohol is the *liver*. The capacity of this organ for holding active substances in its cellular parts is one of its marked physiological distinctions. In instances of poisoning by arsenic, antimony, strychnine, and other poisonous compounds, we turn to the liver, in conducting our analyses, as if it were the central depôt of the foreign matter. It is, practically, the same in respect of alcohol. The liver of the confirmed alcoholic is probably never free from the influence of the poison; it is too often saturated with it.

The effect of the alcohol upon the liver is upon the minute membranous or capsular structure of the organ, upon which it acts to prevent the proper dialysis and free secretion. The organ at first becomes large from the distention of its vessels, the surcharge of fluid matter and the thickening of tissue. After a time there follow contraction of membrane, and slow shrinking of the whole mass of the organ in its cellular parts. Then the shrunken, hardened, roughened mass is said to be " hobnailed," a common but expressive term. By the time this change occurs, the body of him in whom it is developed is usually dropsical in its lower parts, owing to the obstruction offered to the returning blood by the veins, and his fate is sealed.

Now and then, in the progress to this extreme

change and deterioration of tissue, there are intermediate changes. From the blood, rendered pre-
ternaturally fluid by the alcohol, there may tran-
sude, through the investing membrane, plastic
matter which may remain, interfering with natural
function, if not creating active mischief. Again,
under an increase of fatty substance in the body,
the structure of the liver may be charged with
fatty cells, and undergo what is technically designated fatty degeneration. I touch with the lightest
hand upon these deteriorations, and I omit many
others. My object is gained if I but impress you
with the serious nature of the changes that, in this
one organ alone, follow an excessive use of alcohol.

In the course of the early stages of deterioration
of function of the liver from organic change of
structure, another phenomenon, leading speedily
to a fatal termination, is sometimes induced. This
new malady is called diabetes, and consists in the
formation in enormous quantity within the body
of glucose or grape sugar, which substance has to
be eliminated by dialysis, through the kidneys—
often a fatal elimination. The injury causing this
disease through the action of alcohol may possibly
be traced back to an influence upon the nervous
matter; but the appearance of the phenomenon is
coincident with the derangement of the liver, and I
therefore refer to it in this place.

The *kidney*, in like manner with the liver, suffers
deterioration of structure from the continued influence of alcoholic spirit. Its minute structure undergoes fatty modifications; its vessels lose their due
elasticity and power of contraction; or its mem-

branes permit to pass through them that colloidal part of the blood which is known as albumen. This last condition reached, the body loses power as if it were being gradually drained even of its blood. For this colloidal albumen is the primitively dissolved fluid out of which all the other tissues are, by dialytical processes, to be elaborated. In its natural destination it has to pass into and constitute every colloidal part.

The *lungs* do not escape the evil influence that follows the persistent use of alcohol. They, indeed, probably suffer more than we at present know from the acute evils imposed by this agent. The vessels of the lungs are easily relaxed by alcohol; and as they, of all parts, are most exposed to vicissitudes of heat and cold, they are readily congested when, paralysed by the spirit, they are subjected to the effects of a sudden fall of atmospheric temperature. Thus, the suddenly fatal congestions of lungs which so easily befall the confirmed alcoholic during severe winter seasons.

Alcoholic Phthisis; or, The Consumption of Drunkards.

There are yet other and more prolonged, and more certainly fatal mischiefs induced in the lungs by the persistent resort to alcohol; and to one of these I would direct special attention. It is that deterioration of lung tissue to which, in the year 1864, I gave originally the name of *alcoholic phthisis*, or the *consumption of drunkards*. The facts were elicited at first in this manner. In a public hospital to which I acted as physician, I had brought before me, in the course of many years, two thousand persons who were stricken with consumption. I gathered the history of the lives of these, and of the reasons why they had passed into the all but hopeless malady from which they suffered. In my analysis of these histories I found that the leading causes of the malady were, in the great majority of instances, predisposition from hereditary taint; exposure to impure air; want; or certain other allied causes. But the analysis being conducted rigidly, I discovered that, when every individual instance had been classified as due to the causes stated above, there remained thirty-six persons, or nearly two per cent., who were excluded from them, who appeared to suffer purely from the effects of alcohol, and in whom the consumption had been brought into existence by the use of alcohol.

The added observations of eleven years, since the above named fact was recorded in the *Social Science Review*, as a new fact in the history of the disease, have only served to prove, in the minds of other men as well as my own, the truth of the record.

The persons who succumb to this deterioration of structure induced by alcohol are not the exceedingly young, neither are they the old. They are usually over twenty-eight and under fifty-five. The average age may be taken as forty-eight. They are persons of whom it is never expected that their death will be from consumption; and they are generally males. They are probably considered very healthy;—men who can endure anything, sit up late at night, run the extreme of amusements, and yet get through a large amount

of business. They sleep well, eat pretty well, and
drink very well. They are often men of excellent
build of body, and of active minds and habits.
They are not a class of drinkers of strong drinks
who sleep long, take little exercise, and grow
heavy, waxy, pale—

" Sleek-headed men and such as sleep o' nights."

On the contrary, they take moderate rest, and see
as much as they can. Neither in the ordinary
sense are they drunkards: they may never have
been intoxicated in the whole course of their lives;
but they partake freely of any and every alcoholic
drink that comes in their way, and they bear alcohol with a tolerance that is remarkable to observers. They are hard drinkers as distinguished
from sots. Beer is to them as water, wine is weak;
the only thing that upsets them is stiff grog in re-
lays, or a mixture of spirituous drinks carried to
the extent of what they call, in grim joke—in which
death surely joins—" piling the agony."

As a rule these cannot live in what they consider
to be comfort without a daily excess of alcohol,
which excess must needs be renewed on emer-
gencies, if there be greater amount of work to be
done, less sleep to be secured, or more life to be
lived.

As specimens of animal build these persons are
often models of organic symmetry and power. In
fact they resist the enemy they court for so long a
time because of the perfection of their organisation. More than half of those whom I have seen
stricken down with alcoholic phthisis have said

that they had never had a day's illness in their lives
before; but questioned closely it was found that
none of them had actually been quite well. Some
of them had suffered from gout; others from rheu-
matism or neuralgia. They had felt severely any
depression such as that which arises from a cold,
and if they had been subjected suddenly to causes
of excitement or exhaustion, they had detected,
without actually realising its full meaning, that
their balance of power against weakness was reduced, that the end of the beam called strength
was rising, and that an extra quantity of alcohol
was required to bring back equilibrium. As a rule
men of this class are thoughtless of their own
health and their own prospects, for they have an
abundant original store of energy. They are designated as "happy-go-lucky" men, or as men who
"always fall on their feet," which truly they do,
but not without injury.

The countenance of the alcoholic consumptive
differs from that which is usually considered the
countenance of the consumptive person, and
equally from that which all the world adjudges as
belonging to the man who indulges freely in strong
drink. Who does not remember the wan, pale,
sunken check of the youth on whom ordinary consumption has set its mark? And who, again, does
not recall the *facies alcoholica*—the blotched skin,
the purple-red nose, the dull, protruding eye, the
vacant stare of the confirmed sot? The alcoholic
consumptive has none of these characteristics.
His face is the best part of him in all his history.
When his muscles have lost their power, and his

clothes hang loosely on his shrunken limbs, he is
still of fair proportion in the face ; he has little pallor, and he is expressive in feature, so that his
friends are apt to be deceived and to believe that
there must be hope for his recovery, even when
he is beyond every hope.   I remember being actually taken aback on one occasion on finding, in a
man who seemed, from his face, to be in perfect
health, complete destruction of his lungs from the
encroachments of disease ; and I cannot be sur-
prised, therefore, that others, less informed, should
share in such an imperception of danger when it
is close at hand.   Nobody, in a word, " pities the
looks " of these sufferers, and good eyes are necessary to learn that pity is called for.

The phenomena are not always developed at a
time when the sufferer from them is indulging
most freely in alcohol.   On the contrary, it is by no
means uncommon that the habit of excessive indulgence has been stopped for some time previously to
their development.   The reasons assigned by the
patients for abstinence vary.   One man may have
been strongly advised by his friends to desist, or
may himself have undergone a certain measure of
reform ; another has been led by the reading or
hearing of arguments on temperance ; a third, by
want of means to obtain the indulgence ; but by far
the larger number tell you that a time came when
the desire for so much drink did not occur to them.
They will state that they tried the round of the
various spirits, but found that none agreed with
them as before, so that at last they were driven to
rely on beer as the only drink they cared for. We

read all this off clearly enough from a physiological point of view. We see that, in fact, the body
has been resisting the alcohol; that it could not
do away with it as it did when all the excreting
organs were in their full prime; and that those
drinks only can be borne in which the amount of
alcohol is least. But the sufferer does not com-
prehend the fact, and therefore he not unfrequently
concludes that his increasing languor and debility
are due to the necessary withdrawal of the stimulus on which he seems to have been actually feeding during the greater part of his life.

The signs which first indicate failure of health
are usually those of acute pleurisy. There is pain
in the side, quick, sharp, starting. The term
"stitch" in the side is commonly applied to this
pain, and is expressive enough. After a time the
pain becomes continuous, and when it subsides,
suppressed breathing, or difficulty of filling the
chest, is at once felt and recognised. This difficulty is due to the circumstance that a portion of
lung has become adherent to the inner surface of
the chest. The next sign indicating that the
disease (consumption) is present, is, usually, vomiting of blood. In two-thirds of the examples to
which my attention has been directed this has
been the sign that has first caused serious alarm,
and it is commonly on such event that the physician is called in, who examines the chest with the
stethoscope, and finds too often a condition that
is hopeless. From the appearance of that sign
all is—down, down, down towards the grave.

There is no form of consumption so fatal as that

from alcohol. Medicines affect the disease very little, the most judicious diet fails, and change of air accomplishes but slight real good. The sick man with this consumption may linger longer on the highway to dissolution than does his younger companion, but there is this difference between them, that the younger companion may possibly find a by-path to comparative health, while the other never leaves it, but struggles on straight to the fatal end. In plain terms, there is no remedy whatever for alcoholic phthisis. It may be delayed in its course, but it is never cured, and not unfrequently instead of being delayed it runs on to a final termination more rapidly than is common in any other type of the disorder.

The origin of this series of changes from alcohol is again from the membranes. The course of it is through the membranous tissues. The vessels give way after a severe congestive condition, and blood is exuded, or extravasated into the lung. These conditions lead to the destruction of the substance of the pulmonary organs, upon which, and upon the organic changes that follow such destruction, the acute symptoms of the malady under consideration, become quickly and fatally pronounced.

Alcoholic Disease of the Heart.

The heart, not less than the rest of the vital parts, is subjected to deterioration of structure from alcohol. We need not wonder at this when we recall the strain to which it is subjected by the agent, the excess of work it is made to perform. I touched on the mechanical evils that befall the heart from these circumstances in my last lecture, and the structural evils which I have now to specify are not less grave. The membranous structures which envelope and line the organ are changed in quality, are thickened, rendered cartilaginous, and even calcareous or bony. Then the valves, which are made up of folds of membrane, lose their suppleness, and what is called valvular disease is permanently established. The coats of the great blood-vessel leading from the heart, the aorta, share, not unfrequently, in the same changes of structure, so that the vessel loses its elasticity and its power to feed the heart by the recoil from its distention, after the heart, by its stroke, has filled it with blood.

Again, the muscular structure of the heart fails, owing to degenerative changes in its tissue. The elements of the muscular fibre are replaced by fatty cells; or if not so replaced are themselves transferred into a modified muscular texture in which the power of contraction is greatly reduced.

Those who suffer from these organic deteriorations of the central and governing organ of the circulation of the blood learn the fact so insidiously, it hardly breaks upon them until the mischief is far advanced. They are, for years, conscious of a central failure of power from slight causes, such as over-exertion, trouble, broken rest, or too long abstinence from food. They feel what they call a "sinking," but they know that wine or some other stimulant will at once relieve the sensation. Thus they seek to relieve it until at last they discover that the remedy fails. The jaded, over-worked, faithful heart will bear no more; it has run its course, and, the governor of the blood stream broken, the current either overflows into the tissues, gradually damming up the courses, or under some slight shock or excess of motion ceases at the centre.

Other Organic Changes.

In the eyeball certain colloidal changes take place from the influence of alcohol, the extent of which have as yet been hardly thought of, certainly not in any degree studied, as in future they will be. We have learned of late years that the crystalline lens, the great refracting medium of the eyeball, may, like other colloids, be rendered dense and opaque, by processes which disturb the relationship of the colloidal substance and its water. By this means even the lens of the living eye can be rendered opaque, and the disease called cataract can be artificially produced. Sugar and many salts in excess, in the blood, will lead to this perversion of structure, and after a long time alcohol acting in the manner of salt is capable, in excess, of causing the same modification of the eyeball. Moreover, alcohol injures the delicate nervous expanse upon which the image of all objects we look at is first impressed. It interferes with the vascular supply of this surface, and it leads to changes of structure which are indirectly destructive to the perfect sense of sight.

In yet another mode alcohol perverts the animal

mechanism. By some as yet obscurely definable interference with the natural transmutation of the colloidal substances into saline or crystalloidal, it gives rise to the production of an excess of some salines which appear in the fluid renal secretion. These saline matters accumulated in the blood from inability of the excreting organs to dispose of them, are directly injurious, and exist as possible causes for the promotion of cataractous changes in the crystalline lens and of varied changes in other of the colloidal tissues and membranes. They are also the cause of a disease local in character produced by the aggregation of the saline products, particle by particle, into a compact mass like a stone, or to what is technically called *calculus*. In writing the history of one of the districts of England in which this disease is very prevalent, I expressed many years ago the view that alcoholic indulgence was one of the most telling agencies in the production of the malady. I have seen nothing since that would lead me to alter that statement.

Organic Nervous Lesions from Alcohol.

Lastly, the brain and spinal cord, and all the nervous matter become, under the influence of alcohol, subject, like other parts, to organic deterioration. The membranes enveloping the nervous substance undergo thickening; the blood-vessels are subjected to change of structure, by which their resistance and resiliency is impaired; and the true nervous matter is sometimes modified, by soft-

ening or shrinking of its texture, by degeneration
of its cellular structure, or by interposition of fatty
particles.

These deteriorations of cerebral and spinal matter give rise to a series of derangements, which
show themselves in the worst forms of nervous
disease—epilepsy; paralysis, local or general; insanity.

But not a single serious nervous lesion from alcohol appears without its warning. As a man who,
when drinking at the table, is warned, by certain
unmistakable indications, that the wine is beginning to take decisive effect on his power of expression and motion, so the slow alcoholic is duly
apprised that he is in danger of a more permanent
derangement. He is occasionally conscious of a
failing power of speech; in writing or speaking he
loses common words. He is aware that after
fatigue his limbs are unnaturally weary and heavy,
and he is specially conscious that a sudden fall of
temperature lowers too readily his vital energies.
The worst sign of impending nervous change is
muscular instability, irrespective of the will; that
is to say, an involuntary muscular movement whenever the will is off guard. This is occasionally
evidenced by sudden muscular starts which pass
almost like electrical shocks through the whole of
the body; but it is more frequently and determinately shown in persistent muscular movements
and starts at the time of going to sleep. The volition then is resigned to the overpowering slumber,
and naturally all muscular movement, except the
movement of the heart and of the breathing, should

rest with the will. But now this beautiful order is disturbed. In the motor centres of the nervous organisation the foreign agent is creating disturbance of function. The fact is communicated to the muscles by the nervous fibres, and the active involuntary start of the lower limbs rouses the sleeper in alarm. Ignorant óf the import of these messages of danger, the habituated alcoholic continues too frequently his way, until he finds the agitated limbs unsteady, wanting in power of co-ordinated movement—paralysed.

Deeply interesting as these phenomena from alcohol are, I must leave them here, omitting many others equally significant and equally plain, when they are once pointed out, even to the unprofessional mind. Let it be understood that in each description I have recorded only what alcohol can physically do to the animal economy. It is not always the cause of all or any of these phenomena. They may be induced by other influences and other agents, but it is an agency capable of effecting them, and it is actively employed in the work.

ON SOME OF THE MENTAL PHENOMENA INDUCED BY ALCOHOL.

The purely physical action of alcohol has been so far treated upon in the preceding pages. To that must now be added a few sentences on the influence this agent exerts over the mental functions. Of course such influence is actually manifested by and through physical means, but as yet these are not sufficiently clear to enable us to trace out the mental aberration through the physical process that has led to it. It is better therefore and simpler to treat the present subject in the mere abstract, passing from the agent to its results, without reference to the intermediate line of connection between cause and effect. These mental phenomena in the chronic phase, correspond to the phenomena which belong to the second and third stages of acute alcoholic intoxication.

Loss of Memory or Speech.

One of the first effects of alcohol upon the nervous system in the way of alienation from the natural mental state, is shown in loss of memory. This extends even to forgetfulness of the commonest of things; to names of familiar persons, to dates, to duties of daily life. Strangely too, this failure, like that which indicates, in the aged, the era of second childishness and mere oblivion, does not extend to the things of the past, but is confined to events that are passing. On old memories the mind retains its power; on new ones it requires constant prompting and sustainment.

If this failure of mental power progress, it is followed usually with loss of volitional power. The muscles remain ready to act, but the mind is incapable of stirring them into action. The speech fails at first, not because the mechanism of speech is deficient, but because the cerebral power is insufficient to call it forth to action. The man is reduced to the condition of the dumb animal. Aristotle says, grandly, animals have a voice; man speaks. In this case the voice remains, the speech is lost ; the man sinks to the lower spheres of the living creation, over which he was born to rule.

The failure of speech indicates the descent still deeper to that condition of general paralysis in which all the higher faculties of mind and will are powerless, and in which nothing remains to show the continuance of life except the parts that remain under the dominion of the chain of organic or vegetable nervous matter. Our asylums for the insane are charged with these helpless specimens of humanity. The membranes of the nervous centres of thought and volition have lost, in these, the dialysing function. In some instances, though less frequently than might be supposed, the nervous matter itself is modified, visibly, in texture. The result is the complete wreck of the nervous mechanism, the utter helplessness of will, the absolute dependence upon other hands for the very food that has to be borne to the mouth. The picture is one of breathing death ; of final and perpetual dead intoxication.

Dipsomania.

A second effect of alcohol on the mental organisation is the production of that craving for its incessant supply to which we give the name of dipsomania. In those who are affected with this form of alcoholic disease, a mixed madness and insanity is established, in which the cunning of the mind

alone lives actively, with the vices that ally themselves to it. The arrest of nervous function is partial, and does not extend to the motor centres so
determinately as to those of the higher reasoning
faculties. But, the end, though it may be slow, is
certain, and the end is, as a rule, that general paralysis which I have just described. The dipso-
maniac is, however, capable of recovery, within
certain limits, on one and only one condition, that
the cause of his disease be totally withheld.

Mania a Potu.

The effect of alcohol on the mental functions is
shown in yet another picture of modern humanity
writhing under its use. I mean in the form of
what may be called intermittent indulgence to
dangerous excess. This form of disease has been
named the *mania a potu*, and it is one of the most
desperate of the alcoholic evils. The victims of this
class are not habitual drunkards or topers, but at
sudden intervals they madden themselves with the
spirit; they repent; reform; get a new lease of
life; relapse. In intervals of repentance they are
worn with remorse and regret; in the intervals of
madness they are the terrible members of the community. In their furious excitement they spread
around their circle the darkness of desolation, fear,
and despair. Their very footsteps carry dread to
those who, most helpless and innocent, are under
their fearful control. They strike their dearest
friends; they strike themselves. Retaining suffi-

cient nervous power to wield their limbs, yet not sufficient to guide their reason, they become the dangerous alcoholic criminals whom our legislators, fearing to touch the cause of their malady, would fain try to cure by scourge and chain.

To us physiologists these " maniacs a potu " are men under the experiment of alcohol, with certain of their brain centres (which I could fairly define if the present occasion were befitting) paralysed, and with a broken balance, therefore, of brain power, which we, with infinite labor and much exactitude, have learned to understand. Our remedy for such aberration of nervous function, if we were legislators, would be simple enough. We should not whip the maniac back again to the drink; we should try to break up the evil by taking the drink from the maniac. But then we are only physiologists. We have nothing to do with that £117,000,000 of invested capital, and we are not practical in reference to it.

TRANSMITTED DISEASE.

The most solemn fact of all bearing upon these mental aberrations produced by alcohol, and upon the physical not less than the mental, is, that the mischief inflicted on man by his own act and deed cannot fail to be transferred to those who descend from him, and who are thus irresponsibly afflicted. Amongst the many inscrutable designs of nature none is more manifest than this, that physical vice, like physical feature and physical virtue, descends

in line.   It is, I say, a solemn reflection for every
man and every woman, that whatever we do to
ourselves so as to modify our own physical con-
formation and mental type, for good or for evil, is
transmitted to generations that have yet to be.

Not one of the transmitted wrongs, physical or
mental, is more certainly passed on to those yet
unborn than the wrongs which are inflicted by
alcohol.   We, therefore, who live to reform the
present age in this respect, are stretching forth
our powers to the next; to purify it, to beautify it,
and to lead it toward that millennial happiness and
blessedness, which, in the fulness of time, shall visit
even the earth, making it, under an increasing light
of knowledge, a garden of human delight, a Para-
dise regained.

SUMMARY.

In summary of what has past, I may be brief-
ness itself.

This chemical substance, alcohol, an artificial
product devised by man for his purposes, and in
many things that lie outside his organism a useful
substance, is neither a food nor a drink suitable for
his natural demands.   Its application as an agent
that shall enter the living organization is properly
limited by the learning and skill possessed by the
physician—a learning that itself admits of being
recast and revised in many important details, and
perhaps in principles.

If this agent do really for the moment cheer the
weary and impart a flush of transient pleasure to

the unwearied who crave for mirth, its influence (doubtful even in these modest and moderate degrees) is an infinitesimal advantage, by the side of an infinity of evil for which there is no compensation, and no human cure.

APPENDIX.

I. REFERENCES TO TABLES.

TABLE I.

NAMES OF ANCIENT ROMAN WINES.

1	4	6
Falernum	Vetus	Cnidum
Massicum	Novum	Adrium
Setinum	Recens	
Surrentinum	Hornum	7
	Trimum	
2	Molle	Mustum
Chium	Lene	Protropum
Lesbium	Vetustate edentulum	Mulsum
Leucadium	Asperum	Sapa
Naxium	Calenum	Defrutum
Mamertinum	Cœcubum	Carenum
Thasium	Albanum	
Mœnium	Merum	8
Mareoticum	Fortius	
		Passum
3	5	Passum creticum
Album	Coum	
Nigrum	Rhodium	9
Rubrum	Myndian	
	Halicarnassum	Murrhina

TABLE II.

WINES OF ITALY.

Vesuvius.

Vino Greco
Mangiaguerra
Verracia
Vino Vergine

Tuscany.

Florence (white and red)
Monte Pulciano
Montalneo
Porte Hercole

Lombardy.

Modenese
Montserrat
Marcemino
Brescian
Veronese
Placentine
Lumelline
Pucine

Naples.

Campania or Pausilippo
Muscatel
Surentine
Salerpitan
Chiarello
Carcassone
Lachryma Christi
Albano
Montefiascone

Nomentan
Monteran
Velitrin
Prænetic
Il Romanesca
D'Orvieto

Sicilian, Sardinian, and Corsican.

Catanean
Panormitan
Messinian
Syracusan

Genoa.

Vino di Monte Vernaccia
Vino Tinto
Madeira

WINES OF MADEIRA AND CANARIES ISLANDS.

Madeira Sec
Canary or Palm Sec

WINES OF FRANCE AND SWITZERLAND.

Languedoc
Picardy
Champagne
Burgundy
Vino Amabile, or Vino di Cinque Terre
Vino Razzese
Muscadine

TABLE II.—*Continued.*

Rosatz
Vino Piccante

WINES OF GERMANY.

Tyrolese Tramin
Etsch
Wine of Worms
Edinghof
Ambach
Rhenish
Mayne
Moselle
Neckar
Elsass
Hock
Bohemian
Silesian
Thuringian
Misnian
Naumberg
Brandenburg

WINES OF AUSTRIA AND HUNGARY.

Klosterneuberg
Brosenberg

Edenburg
Tokay

WINES OF SPAIN AND PORTUGAL.

Aland
Alicant
Sherry (or Xeres)
Spanish Malmsey
Tarragan
Salamanca
Malaga
Cordova
Galicia
Andalusia
Vino de Toro
Spanish
Vin de Beaune (or Partridge eye)
Cote Roti
St. Laurence
Frontiniac
Muscat de Lion
Cahors
Hermitage
Grave
Vin d'Haye

Neufchatel
Velteline
Lacote
Reiff

TABLE III.

TABLE OF THE CONTENTS OF DIFFERENT WINES IN A QUART
OF EACH.

	Highly Rectified Spirit.			Thick, Unctuous Resinous Matter.			Gummy and Tartareous Matter.			Water.			
	oz.	dr.	gr.	oz.	dr.	gr.	oz.	dr.	gr.	lbs.	oz.	dr.	gr.
Aland	1	6	0	3	2	0	1	5	0	2	5	3	0
Alicant . . .	3	6	0	6	0	20	0	1	40	2	2	6	0
Burgundy . . .	2	2	0	0	4	0	0	1	40	2	9	0	20
Carcassone . . .	2	6	0	0	4	10	0	1	20	2	8	4	30
Champagne . .	2	5	20	0	6	40	0	1	0	2	8	3	0
French	3	0	0	0	6	40	0	1	0	2	8	0	20
Frontignac . . .	3	0	0	3	4	0	0	5	20	2	4	6	30
Vin Grave . . .	2	0	0	0	6	0	0	2	0	2	9	0	0
Hermitage . . .	2	7	0	1	2	0	0	1	40	2	7	5	20
Madeira	2	3	0	3	2	0	2	0	0	2	4	3	0
Malmsey . . .	4	0	0	4	3	0	2	3	0	2	1	2	0
Vino di Monte Pulciano . .	2	6	0	0	3	0	0	2	40	2	8	0	20
Moselle	2	2	0	0	4	20	0	1	30	2	9	0	10
Muscadine . . .	3	0	0	2	4	0	1	0	0	2	5	4	0
Neufchatel . . .	3	2	0	4	0	0	1	7	0	2	2	7	0
Palm Sec . . .	2	3	0	2	4	0	4	4	0	2	2	5	0
Pontack	2	0	0	0	5	20	0	2	20	2	9	0	40
Old Rhenish . .	2	0	0	1	0	0	0	2	20	2	8	5	40
Rhenish	2	2	0	0	3	20	0	1	34	2	9	1	6
Salamanca . . .	3	0	0	3	4	0	2	0	0	2	3	4	0
Sherry	3	0	0	6	0	0	2	2	0	2	0	6	0
Spanish	1	2	0	2	4	0	9	4	0	1	10	6	0
Vino Tinto . . .	3	0	0	6	4	0	1	6	0	2	0	6	0
Tokay	2	2	0	4	3	0	5	0	0	2	0	3	0
Tyrol Red Wine .	1	4	0	1	2	0	0	4	0	2	8	6	0
Red Wine . . .	1	6	0	0	4	40	0	2	0	2	9	3	20
White	2	0	0	0	7	0	0	3	0	2	7	0	0

TABLE IV.

LIST OF SUBSTANCES THAT WILL PRODUCE ANÆSTHETIC SLEEP.

Nitrous oxide gas

Carbonic oxide gas

Carbonic acid gas

Bisulphide of carbon

Light carburetted hydrogen (hydride of methyl or marsh gas)

Methylic alcohol

Methylic ether gas

Chloride of methyl gas

Bichloride of methylene

Terchloride of formyl, or chloroform

Tetra-chloride of carbon

Heavy carburetted hydrogen gas (olefiant gas or ethylene)

Ethylic or absolute ether

Chloride of ethyl

Bichloride of ethylene (Dutch liquid)

Bromide of ethyl, or hydrobromic ether

Hydride of amyl

Amylene

Benzol

Turpentine spirit

TABLE V.

ALCOHOLS.

Elementary Composition.

Methylic or Protylic (wood spirit) . .	$C\ \ H_3\ \ HO$
Ethylic or Deutylic (common alcohol) .	$C_2\ \ H_5\ \ HO$
Propylic or Trilylic	$C_3\ \ H_7\ \ HO$
Butylic or Tetrylic	$C_4\ \ H_9\ \ HO$
Amylic or Pentylic (potato spirit, fusel oil) .	$C_5\ \ H_{11}\ \ HO$
Hexylic	$C_6\ \ H_{13}\ \ HO$
Heptylic or Œnanthic	$C_7\ \ H_{15}\ \ HO$
Octylic	$C_8\ \ H_{17}\ \ HO$
Decatylic	$C_{10}\ \ H_{21}\ \ HO$
Cetylic	$C_{16}\ \ H_{33}\ \ HO$
Melylic	$C_{30}\ \ H_{61}\ \ HO$

TABLE VI.

RADICALS OF ALCOHOLS.

Composition.	Old name.	New name.
C H$_3$	Methyl	Protylen.
C$_2$ H$_6$	Ethyl	Deutylen.
C$_3$ H$_7$	Propyl	Tritylen.
C$_4$ H$_9$	Butyl	Tetrylen.
C$_5$ H$_{12}$	Amyl	Pentylen.
C$_6$ H$_{13}$	Hexyl	Hexylen.
C$_7$ H$_{15}$	Heptyl	Heptylen.
C$_8$ H$_{17}$	Octyl	Octylen.
C$_{10}$ H$_{21}$	Decatyl	—
C$_{16}$ H$_{33}$	Cetyl	—
C$_{30}$ H$_{61}$	Melyl	—

TABLE VII.

ALCOHOLS.

Name.		Chemical composition.	Vapor density.	Specific gravity.	Boiling point.	
Old.	New.		H$_2$ = 1.	Water 1000.	Cen.	Fah.
Methylic	Protylic .	C H$_4$ O	16	814 at 0″ C	60	140
Ethylic .	Deutylic	C$_2$ H$_6$ O	23	792 "	78	172
Butylic .	Tetrylic .	C$_4$ H$_{10}$ O	37	803 "	110	230
Amylic .	Pentylic	C$_5$ H$_{12}$ O	44	811 "	132	270

TABLE VIII.

Alcohols.	Aldehydes.	Acids.
Mythylic C H_4 O	Formaldehyde . C H_2 O	Formic . C H_2 O_2
Ethylic . C_2 H_6 O	Aldehyde . . . C_2 H_4 O	Acetic . C_2 H_4 O_2
Propylic C_3 H_8 O	Propionaldehyde C_3 H_6 O	Proponic C_3 H_6 O_2
Butylic . C_4 H_{10} O	Butylaldehyde . C_4 H_8 O	Butyric . C_4 H_8 O_2
Amylic . C_5 H_{12} O	Valeraldehyde . C_5 H_{10} O	Valerianic C_5 $H_{10}O_2$

TABLE IX.

ETHERS.

NAME.	Composition.	Form.	Boiling point.
Methyl Ether . .	C_2 H_6 O	Gas	. .
Ethyl " . . .	C_4 H_{10} O	Fluid	94° Fah.
Propyl " . . .	C_6 H_{14} O	"	153° Fah.
Butyl " . . .	C_8 H_{18} O	"	219° Fah.
Amyl " . . .	C_{10} H_{22} O	"	348° Fah.

TABLE X.

CHLORIDES.

NAME.		Chemical composition.	Vapor density.	Specific gravity.	Boiling point.	
Old.	New.		$H_2 = 1$.	Water 1000.	Cen.	Fah.
Methyl .	Protyl .	C H_3 Cl	25	Gas	. .	. .
Ethyl .	Deutyl.	C_2 H_5 Cl	32	921 at 0″ C.	11	52
Butyl .	Tetryl .	C_4 H_9 Cl	46	880 "	70	158
Amyl .	Pentyl .	C_5 H_{11} Cl	53	. .	102	216

TABLE XI.

IODIDES.

NAME.		Chemical composition.	Vapor density.	Specific gravity.	Boiling point.		Per cent. of Iodine.
Old.	New.		$H_2 = 1.$	Water 1000.	Cen.	Fah.	
Methyl	Protyl	$C\ H_3\ I$	71	2240	42	108	89.4
Ethyl .	Deutyl	$C_2\ H_5\ I$	78	1946	72	162	81.4
Butyl .	Tetryl	$C_4\ H_9\ I$	92	1604	120	248	69.0
Amyl .	Pentyl	$C_6\ H_{11}\ I$	99	1511	146	295	64.1

TABLE XII.

NITRITES.

NAME.		Chemical composition.	Vapor density.	Specific gravity.	Boiling point.	
Old.	New.		$H_2 = 1.$	Water 1000.	Cen.	Fah.
Methyl .	Protyl .	$C\ H_3\ N\ O_2$	30	..	..	..
Ethyl .	Deutyl .	$C_2\ H_5\ N\ O_2$	37	0.917	18	64
Butyl .	Tetryl .	$C_4\ H_9\ N\ O_2$	51	..	64	147
Amyl .	Pentyl .	$C_8\ H_{11}\ N\ O_2$	58	0.877	96	205

II. REFERENCES TO WORDS AND DERIVATIONS.

While the delivery of these Lectures was in progress, I received from John F. Stanford, Esq., M.A., F.R.S., a philological scholar, whose dictionary of Anglicised foreign words and phrases will, it is to be hoped, soon appear— many very useful and interesting notes relating to derivations of words and terms respecting alcohol. By his kind permission I add a few of his notes in this place.

Alcohol.—The best Arabic scholars write the word Al-Kool, though there is no word in Arabic which corresponds to the meaning assigned to it in the English language.

Aqua Vitæ.—This word, Mr. Stanford reminds me, is used by Shakspeare.

(*Nurse.*) "Give me some aqua vitæ."—*Romeo and Juliet*, Act. iii. sc. 2.

"I would as soon trust an Irishman with my aqua vitæ bottle."—*Merry Wives of Windsor.*

Aqua vitæ was, Mr. Stanford believes, made before any other spirit, viz., about 1260 A.D., by the monks of Ireland, who got the secret from Spain, the Spaniards having got it from the Moors, and the Moors (Arabs) from the Chinese. Whisky, he thinks, was possibly the oldest term applied to aqua vitæ. The etymon is usige-biatha, which in Erse means aqua vitæ, corrupted afterwards to usquebaugh. This compound term shared the fate of many other words, and was abbreviated to *usige*, whence whisky.

Arrac.—Hindustane for an alcohol, distilled from palm-tree juice and several other juices : it is the aqua vitæ of the East. The word is corrupted to Raki in Russia, Turkey, and Germany, or sometimes to Râkk. The intoxicating liquor made from the juice of the palm-tree is called in India and Ceylon Toddee, whence the Scotch term "Toddy." There is a coarse Arrac called Pariah Arrac, very generally consumed throughout India, which is rendered narcotic by addition of extract of Indian hemp. The importation of Arrac or Rack was regulated by 11 Geo. I. c. 30. It was imported to make punch, so called Rack punch.

Gin.—This term Mr. Stanford traces from French

ginévre, abbreviated from the Italian *ginepro*, Latin *juniperus*, English *juniper*, the berries of the juniper being used in the distillation of the spirit as a flavoring substance.

Gin-sing.—This is the term used by the Chinese for the famous Mandrake narcotic reputed to be worth its weight in gold for medicinal purposes, and at the head of their pharmacopœia.

Metheglin.—Was the name of a fermented honey-drink of Cornwall, an intoxicating narcotic beverage.

Potheen or Poteen—Irish, Poitin.—A small pot or still, the name of the liquor being derived from the still in which it was made. Poitin is probably from the Latin *potio*, a drink.

Rum.—Mr. Stanford believes the word "rum" to be an abbreviation, by aphæresis, of sacca-rum, not an original native name.

PUBLICATIONS

OF THE

National Temperance Society

AND PUBLICATION HOUSE.

THE NATIONAL TEMPERANCE SOCIETY, organized in 1866 for the purpose of supplying a sound and able Temperance literature, have already stereotyped and published *three hundred and fifty* publications of all sorts and sizes, from the one-page tract up to the bound volume of 500 pages. This list comprises books, tracts, and pamphlets, containing essays, stories, sermons, arguments, statistics, history, etc., upon every phase of the question. Special attention has been given to the department

For Sunday-School Libraries.

Over sixty volumes have already been issued, written by some of the best authors in the land. These have been carefully examined and unanimously approved by the Publication Committee of the Society, representing the various religious denominations and Temperance organizations of the country, which consists of the following members:

PETER CARTER,	Rev. J. B. DUNN,
Rev. W. M. TAYLOR,	Rev. A. G. LAWSON,
A. A. ROBBINS,	Rev. ALFRED TAYLOR,
REV. HALSEY MOORE.	R. R. SINCLAIR,
T. A. BROUWER,	Rev. C. D. FOSS,
J. N. STEARNS,	JAMES BLACK,

Rev. WILLIAM HOWELL TAYLOR.

These volumes have been cordially commended by leading clergymen of all denominations, and by various national and State bodies, all over the land.

The following is the list, which can be procured through the regular Sunday-School trade, or by sending direct to the rooms of the Society:

Rev. Dr. Willoughby and his Wine. 12mo, 458 pages. By Mrs. MARY SPRING WALKER, author of "The Family Doctor," etc, . . . **$1 50**

This thrillingly interesting book depicts in a vivid manner the terrible influence exerted by those who stand as the servants of God, and who sanction the social custom of wine-drinking. It is fair and faithful to the truth. It is not a bitter tirade against the church or the ministry. On the contrary, it plainly and earnestly acknowledges that the ministry is the friend of morality, and the great bulwark of practical virtue.

At Lion's Mouth. 12mo, 410 pp. By Miss MARY DWINELL CHELLIS, author of "Temperance Doctor," "Out of the Fire," "Aunt Dinah's Pledge," etc., ... **$1 25**

This is one of the best books ever issued, written in a simple yet thrilling and interesting style. It speaks boldly for the entire suppression of the liquor traffic, depicting vividly its misery and wrongs resulting from it. The Christian tone is most excellent, showing the necessity of God's grace in the heart to overcome temptation and the power of appetite, and the influence which one zealous Christian can exert upon his companions and the community.

Aunt Dinah's Pledge. 12mo, 318 pages. By Miss MARY DWINELL CHELLIS, author of "Temperance Doctor," "Out of the Fire," etc., ... **$1 25**

Aunt Dinah was an eminent Christian woman. Her pledge included swearing and smoking, as well as drinking. It saved her boys, who lived useful lives, and died happy; and by quiet, yet loving and persistent work, names of many others were added who seemed almost beyond hope of salvation.

The Temperance Doctor. 12mo, 370 pages. By Miss MARY DWINELL CHELLIS, ... **$1 25**

This is a true story, replete with interest, and adapted to Sunday-school and family reading In it we have graphically depicted the sad ravages that are caused by the use of intoxicating beverages; also, the blessings of Temperance, and what may be accomplished by one earnest soul for that reform. It ought to find readers in every household.

Out of the Fire. 12mo, 420 pages. By Miss MARY DWINELL CHELLIS, author of "Deacon Sim's Prayers," etc., ... **$1 25**

It is one of the most effective and impressive Temperance books ever published. The evils of the drinking customs of society, and the blessings of sobriety and total abstinence, are strikingly developed in the history of various families in the community.

History of a Threepenny Bit. 18mo, 216 pages, ... **$0 75**

This is a thrilling story, beautifully illustrated with five choice wood engravings. The story of little Peggy, the drunkard's daughter, is told in such a simple yet interesting manner that no one can read it without realizing more than ever before the nature and extent of intemperance, and sympathizing more than ever with the patient, suffering victim. It should be in every Sunday-school library.

Adopted. 18mo, 236 pages. By Mrs. E. J. RICHMOND, author of "The McAllisters," . . . **$0 60**

This book is written in an easy, pleasant yle, seems to be true to nature, true to itself, and withal is full of the Gospel and Temperance.

The Red Bridge. 18mo, 321 pages. By THRACE TALMAN, . . **$0 90**

We have met with few Temperance stories containing so many evidences of decided ability and high literary excellence as this.

The Old Brown Pitcher. 12mo, 222 pages. By the Author of "Susie's Six Birthdays," "The Flower of the Family," etc., **$1 00**

Beautifully illustrated. This admirable volume for boys and girls, containing original stories by some of the most gifted writers for the young, will be eagerly welcomed by the children. It is adapted alike for the family circle and the Sabbath-school library.

Our Parish. 18mo, 252 pages. By Mrs. EMILY PEARSON, . . **$0 75**

The manifold evils resulting from the "still" to the owner's family, as well as to the families of his customers, are truthfully presented. The characters introduced, such as are found in almost every good-sized village, are well portrayed. We can unhesitatingly commend it, and bespeak for it a wide circulation.

The Hard Master. 18mo, 278 pages, By Mrs. J. E. McCONAUGHY, author of "One Hundred Gold Dollars," and other popular Sunday-School books, ... **$0 85**

This interesting narrative of the temptations, trials, hardships, and fortunes of poor orphan boy illustrates in a most striking manner the value of "right principles," especially of honesty truthfulness, and TEMPERANCE.

Echo Bank. 18mo, 269 pages. By ERVIE, ... **$0 85**

This is a well-written and deeply interesting narrative, in which is clearly shown the suffering and sorrow that too often follow and the dangers that attend boys and young men at school and at college, who suppose they can easily take a glass or two occasionally, without fear of ever being aught more than a moderate drinker.

Rachel Noble's Experience. 18mo, 325 pages. By BRUCE EDWARDS. **$0 90**

This is a story of thrilling interest, ably and eloquently told. and is an excellent book for Sunday-school libraries. It is just the book for the home circle, and cannot be read without benefiting the reader and advancing the cause of Temperance.

Gertie's Sacrifice; or Glimpses at Two Lives. 18mo, 189 pages. By Mrs. F. D. GAGE, ... **$0 50**

A story of great interest and power, giving a "glimpse at two lives," and showing how Gertie sacrificed herself as a victim of fashion, custom, and law.

Time will Tell. 12mo, 307 pages. By Mrs. WILSON, . . . **$1 00**

A Temperance tale of thrilling interest and unexceptionable moral and religious tone. It is full of incidents and characters of everyday life, while its lessons are plainly and forcibly set before the reader. The pernicious results of the drinking usages in the family and social circle are plainly set forth.

Philip Eckert's Struggles and Triumphs. 18mo, 216 pages. By the author of "Margaret Clair," **$0 60**

This interesting narrative of a noble, manly boy, in an intemperate home, fighting with the wrong and battling for the right, should be read by every child in the land.

Jug-Or-Not. 12mo, 346 pages. By Mrs. J. McNAIR WRIGHT, author of "John and the Demijohn," "Almost a Nun," "Priest and Nun,"etc., ... **$1 25**

It is one of her best books, and treats of the physical and hereditary effects of drinking in a clear, plain, and familiar style, adapted to popular reading, and which should be read by all classes in the community, and find a place in every Sunday-school library.

The Broken Rock. 18mo, 139 pages. By KRUNA, author of "Lift a Little," etc., ... **$0 50**

It beautifully illustrates the silent and holy influence of a meek and lowly spirit upon the heartless rumseller until the rocky heart was broken.

Andrew Douglass. 18mo, 232 pages, **$0 75**

A new Temperance story for Sunday-schools, written in a lively, energetic, and popular style, adapted to the Sabbath-school and the family circle.

Vow at the Bars. 18mo, 108 pages. **$0 40**

It contains four short tales, illustrating four important principles connected with the Temperance movement, and is well adapted for the family circle and Sabbath-school libraries.

Job Tufton's Rest. 12mo, 332 pages, ... **$1 25**

A story of life's struggles, written by the gifted author, CLARA LUCAS BALFOUR, depicting most skilfully and truthfully many a life-struggle with the demon of intemperance.

Humpy Dumpy. 12mo, 316 pp. By Rev. J. J. DANA, . . . **$1 25**

In this book, a corner grocery is the source of much evil, and a mission-school, by its Christian teachings, the means of rescuing many from the downward path.

Frank Oldfield; or, Lost and Found. 12mo, 408 pages, . . . **$1 50**

This excellent story received the prize of £100 in England, out of eighty-three manuscripts submitted; and by an arrangement with the publishers we publish it in this country with all the original illustrations. It is admirably adapted to Sunday-school libraries.

Tom Blinn's Temperance Society, and other Stories. 12mo, 316 pages, ... **$1 25**

This is the title of a new book written by T. S. ARTHUR, the well-known author of "Ten Nights in a Bar-room," and whose fame as an author should bespeak for it a wide circulation. It is written in Mr. ARTHUR's best style, composed of a series of tales adapted to every family and library in the land.

The Harker Family. 12mo, 336 pages. By EMILY THOMPSON, **$1 25**

A simple, spirited, and interesting narrative, written in a style especially attractive, depicting the evils that arise from intemperance, and the blessings that followed the earnest efforts of those who sought to win others to the paths of total abstinence. Illustrated with three engravings. The book will please all.

Come Home, Mother. 18mo, 143 pages. By NELSIE BROOK. Illustrated with six choice engravings, ... **$0 50**

A most effective and interesting book, describing the downward course of the mother, and giving an account of the sad scenes, but effectual endeavors, of the little one in bringing her mother back to friends, and leading her to God. It should be read by everybody.

Tim's Troubles. 12mo, 350 pages. By Miss M. A. PAULL, . . **$1 50**

This is the second Prize Book of the United Kingdom Band of Hope Union, reprinted in this country with all the original illustrations. It is the companion of "Frank Oldfield," written in a high tone, and will be found a valuable addition to our Temperance literature.

The Drinking Fountain Stories. 12mo, 192 pages, ... **$1 00**

This book of illustrated stories for children contains articles from some of the best writers for children in America, and is beautifully illustrated with forty choice wood engravings.

The White Rose. By Mary J. Hedges. 16mo, 320 pages, . . **$1 25**

The gift of a simple white rose was the means of leading those who cared for it to the Saviour. How it was done is very pleasantly told, also the wrongs resulting in the use of strong drink forcibly shown.

Hopedale Tavern, and What it Wrought. 12mo, 252 pages. By J. WILLIAM VAN NAMEE, . $1 00

It shows the sad results which followed the introduction of a Tavern and Bar in a beautiful and quiet country town, whose inhabitants had hitherto lived in peace and enjoyment The contrast is too plainly presented to fail to produce an impression on the reader, making all more desirous to abolish the sale of all intoxicants.

Roy's Search; or, Lost in the Cars. 12mo, 364 pages. By HELEN C. PEARSON, ... $1 25

This new Temperance book is one of the most interesting ever published—written in a fresh, sparkling style, especially adapted to please the boys, and contains so much that will benefit as well as amuse and interest that we wish all the boys in the land might read it.

How Could He Escape? 12mo, 324 pages. By Mrs. J. McNAIR WRIGHT, author of "Jug-Or-Not." Illustrated with ten engravings, designed by the author, ... $1 25

This is a true tale, and one of the writer's best productions. It shows the terrible effects of even one glass of intoxicating liquor upon the system of one unable to resist its influences, and the necessity of grace in the heart to resist temptation and overcome the appetite for strong drink.

The Best Fellow in the World. 12mo, 352 pages. By Mrs. J. McNAIR WRIGHT, author of "Jug-Or-Not," "How Could He Escape?" "Priest and Nun," $1 25

"The Best Fellow," whose course is here portrayed, is one of a very large class who are led astray and ruined simply because they are such "good fellows." To all such the volume speaks in thrilling tones of warning, shows the inevitable consequences of indulging in strong drink, and the necessity of divine grace in the heart to interpose and save from ruin.

Frank Spencer's Rule of Life. 18mo, 180 pages. By JOHN W KIRTON, author of "Buy Your Own Cherries," "Four Pillars of Temperance," etc., etc., . $0 50

This is written in the author's best style, making an interesting and attractive story for children.

Work and Reward. 18mo, 183 pp. By Mrs. M. A. HOLT, . $0 50

It shows that not the smallest effort to do good is lost sight of by the all-knowing Father, and that faith and prayer must accompany all temperance efforts.

The Pitcher of Cool Water. 18mo, 180 pages. By T. S. ARTHUR, author of "Tom Blinn's Temperance Society," "Ten Nights in a Bar-room," etc., ... $0 50

This little book consists of a series of Temperance stories, handsomely illustrated, written in Mr. ARTHUR's best style, and is altogether one of the best books which can be placed in the hands of children. Every Sunday-school library should possess it.

Little Girl in Black. 12mo, 212 pages. By MARGARET E. WILMER, ... $0 90

Her strong faith in God, who she believes will reclaim an erring father, is a lesson to the reader, old as well as young.

Temperance Anecdotes. 12mo, 288 pages, ... $1 00

This new book of Temperance Anecdotes, edited by GEORGE W. BUNGAY, contains nearly four hundred Anecdotes, Witticisms, Jokes, Conundrums, etc, original and selected, and will meet a want long felt and often expressed by a very large number of the numerous friends of the cause in the land. The book is handsomely illustrated with twelve choice wood engravings.

The Temperance Speaker. By J. N. STEARNS, ... $0 75

The book contains 288 pages of Declamations and Dialogues suitable for Sunday and Day-Schools, Bands of Hope, and Temperance Organizations. It consists of choice selections of prose and poetry, both new and old, from the Temperance orators and writers of the country, many of which have been written expressly for this work.

The McAllisters. 18mo, 211 pages. By Mrs. E. J. RICHMOND, . $0 50

It shows the ruin brought on a family by the father's intemperate habits, and the strong faith and trust of the wife in that Friend above who alone gives strength to bear our earthly trials.

The Seymours. 12mo, 231 pages. By Miss L BATES, . . . $1 00

A simple story, showing how a refined and cultivated family are brought low through the drinking habits of the father, their joy and sorrow as he reforms only to fall again, and his final happy release in a distant city.

Zoa Rodman. 12mo, 262 pages By Mrs. E. J. RICHMOND, $1 00

Adapted more especially to young girls' reading, showing the influence they wield in society, and their responsibility for much of its drinking usages.

Eva's Engagement Ring. 12mo, 189 pages. By MARGARET E. WILMER, author of "The Little Girl in Black," $0 90

In this interesting volume is traced the career of the moderate drinker, who takes a glass in the name of friendship or courtesy.

Packington Parish, and The Diver's Daughter. 12mo, 327 pages. By Miss M. A. PAULL, . . . $1 25

In this volume we see the ravages which the liquor traffic caused when introduced in a hitherto quiet village, and how a minister's eyes were at length opened to its evils, though he had always declared wine to be a "good creature of God," meant to be used in moderation.

Old Times. 12mo. By Miss M. D. CHELLIS, author of "The Temperance Doctor," "Out of the Fire," "Aunt Dinah's Pledge," "At Lion's Mouth," etc., . $1 25

It discusses the whole subject of moderate drinking in the history of a New England village. The incidents, various and amusing, are all facts, and the characters nearly all drawn from real life. The five deacons which figure so conspicuously actually lived and acted as represented.

John Bentley's Mistake. 18mo, 177 pages. By Mrs. M. A. HOLT, $0 50

It takes an important place among our temperance books, taking an earnest, bold stand against the use of cider as a beverage, proving that it is often the first step toward stronger drinks, forming an appetite for the more fiery liquids which cannot easily be quenched.

Nothing to Drink. 12mo, 400 pages. By Mrs. J. McNAIR WRIGHT, author of "The Best Fellow in the World," "Jug-or-Not," "How Could He Escape?" etc., ... $1 50

The story is of light-house keeper and thrilling adventures at sea, being nautical, scientific, and partly statistical, written in a charming, thrilling, and convincing manner. It goes out of the ordinary line entirely, most of the characters being portraits, its scenery all from absolute facts, every scientific and natural-history statement a verity, the sea incidents from actual experience from marine disasters for the last ten years.

Nettie Loring. 12mo, 352 pages. By Mrs. GEO. S. DOWNS, $1 25

It graphically describes the doings of several young ladies who resolved to use their influence on the side of temperance and banish wine from their entertainments, the scorn they excited, and the good results which followed.

The Fire Fighters. 12mo, 294 pages. By Mrs. J. E. McCONAUGHY, author of "The Hard Master," $1 25

An admirable story, showing how a number of young lads banded themselves into a society to fight against Alcohol, and the good they did in the community.

The Jewelled Serpent. 12mo, 271 pages. By Mrs. E. J. RICHMOND, author of "Adopted," "The McAllisters," etc., ... $1 00

The story is written earnestly. The characters are well delineated, and taken from the wealthy and fashionable portion of a large city. The evils which flow from fashionable drinking are well portrayed, and also the danger arising from the use of intoxicants when used as medicine, forming an appetite which fastens itself with a deadly hold upon its victim.

The Hole in the Bag, and Other Stories. By Mrs. J. P. BALLARD, author of "The Broken Rock," "Lift a Little," etc. 12mo, $1 00

A collection of well-written stories by this most popular author on the subject of temperance, inculcating many valuable lessons in the minds of its readers.

The Glass Cable. 12mo, 288 pages. By MARGARET E. WILMER, author of "The Little Girl in Black," "Eva's Engagement Ring," etc., ... $1 25

The style of this book is good, the characters well selected, and its temperance and religious truths most excellent. The moral of the story shows those who sneer at a child's pledge, comparing its strength to a glass cable, that it is in many cases strong enough to brave the storms and temptations of a whole lifetime.

Fred's Hard Fight. 12mo, 334 pages. By Miss MARION HOWARD, ... $1 25

While it shows the trials which a young lad endured through the temptations and enticements offered him by those opposed to his firm temperance and religious principles, and warns the reader against the use of every kind of alcoholic stimulant, it points also to Jesus, the only true source of strength, urging all to accept the promises of strength and salvation offered to every one who will seek it.

The Dumb Traitor. 12mo, 336 pp. By MARGARET E. WILMER, $1 25

Intensely interesting, showing how the prospects of a well-to-do New England family were blighted through the introduction of a box of wine, given in friendship, used as medicine, but proving a dumb traitor in the end.

Esther Maxwell's Mistake. 18mo, 236 pages. By Mrs. E. N. Janvier, author of "Andrew Douglass," $1 00

This book is full of Gospel truth, and written in a simple but earnest style, showing the utter absurdity of endeavoring to forget trouble by the use of strong drink, which Esther, like many others, found soon formed habits not easily broken. Her sudden awakening to this fact, and turning to her Saviour for pardon and help to renounce the temptation to drink, make one of the most touching narratives ever written.

Wealth and Wine. 12mo, 320 pp. By Miss Mary Dwinell Chellis, author of "Temperance Doctor," "At Lion's Mouth," $1 25

This book is written in her best style, showing the deception of the wine-cup and the power of woman's influence, together with the evil influence of social and moderate drinking. Its moral and Christian tone is excellent and none can fail to be profited by its teachings.

The Life Cruise of Captain Bess Adams. 12mo, 413 pages. By Mrs. J. McNair Wright, author of Nothing to Drink, etc., $1 50

A sea-story, filled with thrilling adventures on the deep, and intensely interesting scenes on land in the midst of a quaint old sea-coast town, proving effectually that alcoholic drinks are not needed on shipboard or on land, and should be absolutely banished. The brave Christian character of Captain Adams and the heroism of his daughter, Bess, together with the pure religious tone pervading every page, make this one of the most interesting books ever written.

The Model Landlord. 18mo. By Mrs. M. A. Holt, author of "John Bentley's Mistake," "Work and Reward.". . $0 60

It shows how a "model landlord" who keeps a gilded saloon for fashionable wine-drinkers, though he may attend church, give money to the poor, and circulate in the "first society," may be the greatest instrument in leading the young down to destruction.

Miscellaneous Publications.

The Bases of the Temperance Reform. 12mo, 224 pages. By Rev. Dawson Burns, . . . $1 00

This is an English prize essay, which took the second prize under the liberal offer of James Teare for the best essay on the entire temperance question.

Bacchus Dethroned. 12mo, 248 pages. By Frederick Powell, $1 00

This is an English prize essay, written in response to a prize offered by James Teare, of England, for the best temperance essay. The question is presented in all its phases, physiological, social, political, moral, and religious. It is very comprehensive.

The National Temperance Orator. 12mo, 288 pp. By Miss L. Penney, $1 00

This is issued in response to the many urgent calls for a book similar to the "New Temperance Speaker," used widely throughout the country. Is contains articles by the best temperance writers of the day, poems, recitations, readings, dialogues, and choice extracts from speeches from some of the ablest temperance speakers in the country, for the use of all temperance workers, Lodges, Divisions, Bands of Hope, etc., etc.

Bugle Notes for the Temperance Army. Price, paper covers, 30 cents; boards, ... $0 35

A new collection of Songs, Quartets, and Glees, for the use of all Temperance gatherings, glee clubs, etc., together with the Odes of the Sons of Temperance and Good Templars.

Temperance Chimes. Price, in paper covers, 30 cents, single copies; $25 per hundred. Price, in board covers, 35 cents; per hundred, ... $30 00

A Temperance Hymn and Tune-Book of 128 pages, comprising a great variety of Glees, Songs, and Hymns designed for the use of Temperance Meetings and Organizations, Bands of Hope, Glee Clubs, and the Home Circle. Many of the Hymns have been written expressly for this book by some of the best writers in the country.

Bound Volumes of Sermons, $1 50

Seventeen sermons delivered upon the invitation of The National Temperance Society, and published in the National Series, have all been bound in one volume, making 400 pages of the best temperance matter of the kind ever published. The sermons are by Revs. Henry Ward Beecher, T L. Cuyler, T. De Witt Talmage, J B. Dunn, John Hall, J. P. Newman, J. W. Mears, C. D. Foss, J. Romeyn Berry, Herrick Johnson, Peter Stryker, C. H. Fowler, H. C. Fish, H. W. Warren, S. H. Tyng, and W. M. Taylor.

Text-Book of Temperance. By Dr. F. R. Lees, . . . $1 50

We can also furnish the above book, which is divided into the following parts: 1. Temperance as a Virtue. 2. The Chemical History of Alcohol. 3. The Dietetics of Temperance. 4. The Pathology of Intemperance. 5. The Medical Question. 6 Temperance in Relation to the Bible. 7. Historical. 8. The National Question and the Remedy. 9. The Philosophy of Temperance.

Forty Years' Fight with the Drink Demon. 12mo, 400 pages. By CHARLES JEWETT, M.D., . $1 50

This volume comprises the history of Dr. Jewett's public and private labors from 1826 to the present time, with sketches of the most popular and distinguished advocates of the cause in its earlier stages. It also records the results of forty years' observation, study, and reflections upon the use of intoxicating drinks and drugs, and suggestions as to the best methods of advancing the cause, etc. The book is handsomely bound, and contains illustrated portraits of early champions of the cause.

Drops of Water. 12mo, 133 pages. By MISS ELLA WHEELER, $0 75

A new book of fifty-six Temperance Poems by this young and talented authoress, suitable for reading in Temperance Societies, Lodge Rooms, Divisions, etc. The simplicity of manner, beauty of expression, earnestness of thought, and nobleness of sentiment running through all of them make this book a real gem, worthy a place by the side of any of the poetry in the country.

Bound Volume of Tracts. 500 pages, ... $1 00

This volume contains all the four, eight, and twelve page tracts published by the National Temperance Society, and comprises Arguments, Statistics, Sketches, and Essays, which make it an invaluable collection for every friend of the Temperance Reform.

Bound Volume of Tracts. No. 2. 384 pp., ... $1 00

Containing all the twenty-four and forty-eight page pamphlets and prize essays published by the National Temperance Society since its organization.

Scripture Testimony Against Intoxicating Wine. By REV. WM. RITCHIE, of Scotland, . . $0 60

An unanswerable refutation of the theory that the Scriptures favor the idea of the use of intoxicating wine as a beverage. It takes the different kinds of wines mentioned in the Scriptures, investigates their specific nature, and shows wherein they differ.

Zoological Temperance Convention. By REV. EDWARD HITCHCOCK, D.D., of Amherst College, $0 75

This fable gives an interesting and entertaining account of a Convention of Animals held in Central Africa, and reports the speeches made on the occasion.

Delavan's Consideration of the Temperance Argument and History, $1 50

This condensed and comprehensive work contains Essays and Selections from different authors, collected and edited by EDWARD C. DELAVAN, Esq., and is one of the most valuable text-books on the subject of Temperance ever issued.

Bible Rule of Temperance; or, Total Abstinence from all Intoxicating Drinks. By REV. GEORGE DUFFIELD, D.D., ... $0 60

This is the ablest and most reliable work which has been issued on the subject. The immorality of the us , sale, and manufacture of intoxicating liquors as a beverage is considered in the light of the Scriptures, and the will and law of God clearly presented.

Alcohol: Its Nature and Effects. By CHARLES A. STOREY, M.D., $0 90

This is a thoroughly scientific work, yet written in a fresh, vigorous, and popular style, in language that the masses can understand. It consists of ten lectures carefully prepared, and is an entirely new work by one amply competent to present the subject.

Four Pillars of Temperance. By JOHN W. KIRTON, . . . $0 75

The Four Pillars are, Reason, Science, Scripture, and Experience. The book is argumentative, historical, and statistical, and the facts, appeals, and arguments are presented in a most convincing and masterly manner.

Communion Wine; or, Bible Temperance. By REV. WILLIAM M. THAYER. Paper, 20 cents; cloth, $0 50

An unanswerable argument against the use of intoxicating wine at Communion, and presenting the Bible argument in favor of total abstinence.

Bible Wines; ; or, The Laws of Fermentation and Wines of the Ancients. 12mo, 139 pages. By REV. WM. PATTON, D.D. Paper, 30 cts.; cloth, . . . $0 60

It presents the whole matter of Bible Temperance and the wines of ancient times in a new, clear, and satisfactory manner, developing the laws of fermentation, and giving a large number of references and statistics never before collected, showing conclusively the existence of unfermented wine in the olden time.

Alcohol: Its Place and Power, by JAMES MILLER; and The Use and Abuse of Tobacco, by JOHN LIZARS, ... $1 00

7

www.ingramcontent.com/pod-product-compliance
Lightning Source LLC
Chambersburg PA
CBHW030836270326
41928CB00007B/1077